# Losing Weight
## is a Healing Journey

# Losing Weight
## is a Healing Journey

A womans guide to losing weight naturally

# Katrina Love Senn

I dedicate this book to my husband and best friend

Damien Senn

# Acknowledgements

Firstly, I'd like to acknowledge all the amazing women in my family.

In particular, I would like to say a big thanks to my Mum, Sandra Brunsden who supported me through my health challenges. When I was sick it was my Mum who spoon fed me back to health.

Thanks to my Aunty Rowan. It was Rowan who introduced me to the world of natural healing.

Thanks to my Nana P who has always encouraged me to do what makes me feel happy. Thanks to my Nana B, who taught me to love and respect nature.

Thanks to my sister Melissa who inspires me to follow my creative dreams, as she pursues hers.

Thanks to my mother in law Pauline Senn, my sisters in law Val, Jehanne and Laura and my gorgeous nieces Cosette, Aisling and Caitlin.

I would also like to acknowledge the amazing men in my family too.

Thanks to my ever supportive Dad, Peter Brunsden, a keen vegetable grower and a believer in eating real food.

Thanks to Pop P for your love and support. Thanks to my brother Alister who always encouraged me to explore my intuition and find my spiritual path.

Thanks to my father in law Gary Senn, brothers in law Myles, Mark and Joffa and my little nephews Blake, Kaden and Marco.

Thanks to Yannis, Christine, Julian and Ari from Skyros, Alan and Lucy from Sunflower Retreats and John, Gaia and Maurizio from The Hill that Breathes for all their love and support.

Thanks to my amazing team of proof readers, Sarah-Helena Barmer, Alani Keiser, Anita Johnston, Clare Fielder and Heather Salter.

Thanks also to my dear friends Amanda Smyth, Lee Thomas, Steve Nobel, AK Luthienne, Davide and Esther De Angelis for their constant inspiration.

Thanks to Mary Pachnos my literary agent, for her invaluable guidance and wisdom.

And finally my special thanks and love to Damien Senn, my amazing husband who helped me to shape and craft the ideas in this book.

# Contents

Introduction......................................................................1

**Katrina's Inspirational Weight Loss Story** ........................7

From breakdown to breakthrough....................................8

The problem with dieting.............................................13

A healing approach to losing weight..............................17

**PHASE 1:   Heal Your Body**...........................................**21**

**Chapter One – Food** ........................................................**23**

Rule 1: Eat consciously...............................................24

Rule 2: Eat real foods.................................................30

Rule 3: Substitution not deprivation. ...........................39

Rule 4: Progress not perfection....................................47

**Chapter Two - Exercise**...................................................**55**

Begin with gentle movements.......................................56

The power of walking. ................................................58

Find a form of exercise you love. .................................59

Connect with your breath.............................................62

**Chapter Three - Body** ................................................ **65**

Your body is your barometer. ............................... 66

Self heal through detoxification. ............................ 71

Rest your body. .................................................... 76

Reconnect your body-mind. ................................. 78

**PHASE 2:   Heal Your Mind** ............................... **81**

**Chapter Four - Thoughts** ........................................ **83**

Work with your thoughts. ..................................... 84

Move beyond confusion. ...................................... 89

Notice your self-talk. ........................................... 92

Silence your inner critic. ...................................... 95

Ask better questions. ........................................... 101

Create healing affirmations. ................................ 104

Visualise your success. ........................................ 106

**Chapter Five – Beliefs** .......................................... **109**

The role of beliefs. .............................................. 110

Question your limiting beliefs. ............................. 114

Break free from self sabotage. ............................. 118

Create supportive beliefs. .................................... 120

Reinforce supportive beliefs. ............................... 124

Boost your self-esteem. ....................................... 127

**PHASE 3:  Heal Your Emotions**.......................................**133**

**Chapter Six – Emotional Eating**...............................**135**

What is emotional eating?.......................................136

The 3 layers of emotion. ........................................144

Emotional eating is a symptom. .............................149

The path of emotional eating. ................................154

The path of emotional healing. ..............................160

You can heal emotional eating.................................174

**Chapter Seven – Starting Your Healing Journey** ........**179**

Be willing to change. ..............................................180

Accept where you are...............................................183

Commit to your healing journey. ...........................185

Find your 'BIG why'. ..............................................189

Take responsibility..................................................194

Step out of your 'comfort zone'...............................197

Learn to trust yourself.............................................201

Keep going until you succeed. ...............................204

**Afterword** ...............................................................**209**

**Additional Resources**............................................**211**

# Introduction

*"The most beautiful people we have known are those who have known defeat, known suffering, known struggle, known loss and have found their way out of the depths. These persons have an appreciation, sensitivity and an understanding of life that fills them with compassion, gentleness, and a deep loving concern. Beautiful people do not just happen!"*

*~ Elisabeth Kübler-Ross*

The idea of losing weight permanently for most women, lingers in the realms of pure fantasy.

Sure there seems to be no lack of media attention bestowed upon quick fix techniques, to help you temporarily shift a few pounds. But keep it off for good? Most would wonder if this was even possible.

From my experience, there are two reasons why women experience ongoing problems with their weight. They either;

1. Don't know what to do, or
2. They know what to do but aren't doing it.

Whatever situation you find yourself in right now, this book can help you to lose weight naturally and permanently. It will also help you to heal your body and experience more freedom around food than ever before.

It is filled with practical insights and motivation to keep you focused on achieving the long term weight loss results that you desire.

I want you to know that I'm not a doctor, dietician, nutritionist, psychologist or fitness freak. I don't count calories, weigh myself regularly and I couldn't even tell you the last time I stepped inside a gym.

What I am is a real woman who was open and willing to learn how to use her weight problem as an opportunity for personal growth, deeper self enquiry and healing.

On my own healing journey I managed to navigate through all the confusion and mystery that surrounds the topic of weight loss to lose over 60 pounds. (Just in case you were wondering that's equivalent to around 25 kilograms or about 50 tubs of butter!)

I lost all of my excess weight without dieting, drugs or surgery and have successfully kept it off for over 12 years. I also managed to detoxify my life and heal my body in the process.

*'Losing Weight is a Healing Journey'* is based upon the breakthrough discoveries I made on my own weight loss journey. It also contains key distinctions that I have gathered from over a decade of further study, applied research and exploration into natural health and well being.

Some of the trainings that I have undertaken in this time include Yoga Teacher Training, Massage Therapy, Reiki Healing, Kinesiology, Meta Medicine, Peak Performance Coaching, Emotional Freedom Technique (EFT), Reflexology, Energy work and Neuro Linguistic Programming (NLP).

The book also contains a selection of heart warming stories from women who have experienced real breakthroughs from attending one of my workshops, yoga retreats or private breakthrough healing sessions.

Through my journey of losing weight naturally, I discovered the self worth, respect and love that I had been searching for all along. As with all successful relationships, it is something that continues to deepen and flourish with time. With each year that passes I continue to feel healthier, younger and more vibrantly alive. I'll be sharing more on my weight loss story as we move through the book.

**So what does this book offer?**

*'Losing Weight is a Healing Journey'* offers you an integrative, honouring and healing approach to weight loss that recognises the inherent beauty, wisdom and natural power that is lying dormant within you.

The focus of this book is to help you create the kind of long term weight loss results that you have dreamt about. It will encourage and inspire you to focus upon your personal healing as well as make the lifestyle adjustments necessary to generate a sustainable flow of nourishment and energy for your body, mind and soul.

There is a deeper reason why you are experiencing weight challenges. This book can help guide you to find your own answers by providing the information, inspiration and support to reconnect you back to your body's inner intelligence.

## So what is this book **not** about?

If you are looking for a fad, starvation or yo-yo type of weight loss program created by someone who has never had a weight problem, then this is not the right book for you. This book does not offer a quick fix solution to all of your life's problems. It does not contain any confusing dogma or anything that you need to accept in blind faith.

My weight loss approach is a holistic one that is born out of my own weight loss healing journey. It recognises the fact that every human being is unique and encourages you to connect with and follow the inherent wisdom within your own body.

## So why did I write this book?

I wrote '*Losing Weight is a Healing Journey*' to offer you fresh hope and guidance on your weight loss journey, whilst helping you to break free from the confusion, anxiety and low self esteem experienced by so many women in our society today.

Having personally experienced what it is like to feel overwhelmed and despondent by conflicting and confusing information, I had a deep desire to write a book that is easy to follow and understand.

I want you to benefit from the many hours that I spent searching for real answers on my own weight loss healing journey. I want to pass on knowledge of the things that I have done that worked, as well as the wisdom generated from things that didn't.

The distinctions that I share in this book have been purposefully designed to help you create sustainable long term results. I know all too well how heart breaking it can be to lose weight only to put it all straight back on again.

This book contains many safe, holistic and empowering healing tools that are available to you. Contrary to what you hear in the mainstream media, you do not need to count calories, weigh your food, take diet pills, have your stomach stapled, undergo liposuction, have a lap-band fitted or endure any other form of surgery, deprivation or embarrassment to achieve the kind of weight loss results that you want.

I personally live and breathe everything that you will read about in this book. Many distinctions that I will share with you, you will not hear about from any other source. It is these ideas and principles that made all the difference to my own weight loss healing journey and I know that they will have a positive and powerful impact upon yours too.

**Finding the hidden treasure.**

Buried in the layers of your excess weight are your secret hopes and hidden dreams. While at first it may not seem obvious to peel back the protective physical, mental and emotional layers, what resides beyond this is everything that you've hoped for.

*'Losing Weight is a Healing Journey'* is designed to guide you back to your true self. By having the willingness to start asking different questions, you have the opportunity to receive new and more empowering answers.

As with any journey worth taking, it won't always be easy. There will be days when you will feel deeply challenged. Just know that with each challenge that you confront, you move one step closer to fulfilling your weight loss dreams. Conquering fears and obstacles on your path will make the gifts and the rewards that follow much more worthwhile.

**A healing approach to losing weight.**

My focus is upon inspiring other women to take a healing approach to losing weight. It involves realising that there is a holistic connection between your body, mind and emotions.

This is a total paradigm shift to the yo-yo dieting world that I was unhappily stuck in for many years.

Your external reality is only ever a reflection of your internal world. When you focus upon positively changing your inner world, your outer world will naturally shift to reflect this.

## Getting the most out of this book.

To get the most out of this book I recommend that you read it in its entirety first. This will set you up with a good understanding of the ideas and information contained within it.

As you progress on your own weight loss healing journey, feel free to dip in and out of this book whenever you are seeking deeper insight, inspiration or motivation.

As you read this book, be kind and gentle with yourself. Take time out to honour and appreciate your uniqueness. If you experience any blocks or resistance, just know that life is calling you forward to connect more fully into your personal power.

For best results it is important that you keep your heart and mind open as you read it. When you take a healing approach to losing weight you open the door to living the life you have always dreamed of.

## You can lose weight naturally!

My message to you is really very simple. You can lose weight naturally and permanently without dieting or deprivation. I have achieved it and I know that by incorporating some new distinctions into your life, that you can achieve it too.

I want you to enjoy all the wonderful experiences that life has to offer without having to constantly worry about lingering weight problems.

You deserve...

- To feel happy, healthy, and vibrant from the inside out.
- To create a healthy and loving relationship with your body.
- To live an extraordinary life, while eating food that tastes great and is good for you.

So my simple question to you is, *'Are you ready to break free from frustration and finally create the body and life of your dreams?'*

OK then... let's get started.

# Katrina's Inspirational Weight Loss Story

*"The weight loss journey is a unique opportunity for self acceptance, healing and growth. As you begin to release the heaviness of your life, you will lose weight naturally and permanently, just as I have done."*

*~ Katrina Love Senn*

## From breakdown to breakthrough.

*"This is my weight loss story. It shares my transformation from living with chronic weight problems, fatigue and sickness to experiencing a life filled with radiant health, energy and vitality. May it inspire you to have the courage to embark upon your own weight loss healing journey."*

*~ Katrina Love Senn*

I loved food about as much as I hated exercise.

I had spent the majority of my teenage years battling with my body and self image. By the time I had turned 20, I was already 60 pounds overweight. I had pretty much resigned myself to the fact that none of the available dieting approaches were ever going to work for me and that I was going to be fat forever.

Of course I didn't have the courage to tell anyone else that, it was just one of those things that I preferred to keep quietly to myself.

It wasn't as if I hadn't tried to lose weight using the conventional methods either. I'd really made an effort to shift all those unwanted pounds. I'd read the magazines, counted the calories and followed the advice of the dieting experts. Sadly the results of my endeavours always seemed to adhere to the same sorry story: fleeting short term weight loss, quickly buried beneath even greater weight gain and lower self esteem.

My unsuccessful dieting attempts left me feeling frustrated, confused and even more uncertain about myself. Low energy and daily doses of depression became a regular part of my day to day existence.

Being a sensitive soul, I felt the pain of everyone and everything. I tried my best to deal with my emotions and perceived inadequacies by squashing them down with food. The binge eating episodes that would follow, although providing me with some temporary relief, only ever functioned to deepen my self-loathing.

While I carried on with the very private struggle with my weight, I couldn't help but feel that I was missing out on all the amazing things that normal skinny girls had. I wondered what it would be like to be in a loving relationship, with a partner who could see beyond my extra layers and love and cherish me for who I was.

I also wanted to know what it would be like to move my body freely, dance and be able to wear whatever I wanted to.

I spent countless hours lamenting over what I thought were the big unanswered questions of my life. Questions I would repeatedly ask myself included... *'Why am I so fat?', 'Is it just because I am big boned?', 'Why aren't any of my friends fat?' and 'What's wrong with me?'*

This background chatter constantly spun around in my head. My mind was my misguided master and it did everything it could to control my life through its irrational rules and warped logic.

In my lowest moments I had become so fixated upon my mental and emotional unhappiness that I had totally disconnected from the fact that my body wasn't particularly happy either. I was feeling down for longer periods of time and my number of 'duvet days' increased. I felt like my life force energy had totally burnt out. I still wonder how I managed to even muster the energy to get out of bed and face the overwhelming stress of my daily life.

At the time, I didn't feel as if I had a whole lot of friends I could turn to, so I sought comfort in food. Food was my salvation and the only thing that gave me pleasure.

**And then one day my body completely broke down.**

I was overseas attending a university conference when my body just collapsed. I was rushed back home on the first available flight. My doctor told me that my condition was critical and ordered that I undergo urgent and extensive medical testing.

I spent the next couple of months bed ridden, sleeping for days on end, waking only to be spoon fed by my mother.

When my test results came back, they indicated that I had a major glucose imbalance, a thyroid disorder and adrenal exhaustion amongst other things. Despite this, my doctor said that it was difficult to pin point exactly what was 'wrong' with me.

I was told that these diseases were 'incurable' and that it was in my best interests to commence a program of experimental medication. When I asked how long I would have to take the medicine for, she responded 'possibly for life'.

Alarm bells immediately began to ring in my intuition. After many years of taking prescription drugs and steroids, I was already disillusioned with modern medicine.

For most of my childhood, I had suffered from chronic allergies, asthma and eczema. The medication that I had taken over the years, although temporarily easing my symptoms, hadn't been able to permanently heal me. In fact, whenever I had suggested to my doctors that I didn't think that my medication was working, they would simply change my prescription or increase my dosages.

I was at a cross roads with a big decision to make. Should I follow my doctors' recommendations and trust that modern medicine would be able to offer me some kind of 'miracle cure' or trust in the inherent intelligence of my body to heal naturally?

I politely told my doctor that I needed some time to think about what I wanted to do. As I did, my mother gave me a reassuring and supportive glance.

**Starting my healing journey.**

After careful consideration, I decided to follow my intuition and set off on my own healing journey. Immediately upon making this decision, I experienced an exhilarating rush of both fear and excitement.

I experienced fear because I didn't really know what I was doing. I thought that there was a very real chance that I could get it wrong and perhaps get even sicker. I simultaneously experienced excitement because I was finally creating space in my life to take back responsibility for my health, with a very real possibility of transforming it for the better. I felt ready to allow deeper truths to emerge in my life and to reconnect with my own power.

I have to admit that I was pretty scared. This was all new to me and I felt way out of my depth. I had never done anything like this before. I didn't even know of anyone who had successfully healed themselves using natural methods.

I realized that all I could really do was take a deep breath and step powerfully into the process. I accepted the fact that I wasn't going to have all the answers straight away and I opened myself to trust in the guiding intelligence of the world around me. It was the first time that I had ever trusted in the process of life and in my body.

The decision brought me a deep sense of clarity unlike any that I had ever experienced before. I felt as if I had finally moved into the driver's seat in my own life. It was a wonderful feeling of exhilaration, freedom and adventure.

As I journeyed along I was magically led to many different sources of holistic and natural health information; including books, natural healers and spiritual teachers. My life had finally begun to turn around.

In those early days, my entire focus was on regenerating my health. I discovered an amazing naturopath and healer who was able to help me cleanse and detoxify my body through food and nutrition. She also supported and encouraged me to connect with and open to my creative, sensitive and intuitive nature.

By sheer necessity all the energy that I had previously devoted towards dieting and worrying about my weight was now dedicated towards regaining my health.

With this change in focus my body started to respond very quickly. The more I focused on my own health and inner healing, the more I found my energy, strength and enthusiasm for life returning.


**And then an incredible thing happened.**


After just a couple of months my naturopath noted that not only was my body starting to heal itself but I was also starting to shed my excess weight.

Could you imagine my excitement and surprise when I found out that I was losing weight naturally without any effort whatsoever after so many years of struggle?

I didn't have to go on some crazy starvation diet, take pills or undergo any type of surgery. All I needed to do was follow the wisdom of my body's natural desire to heal and be healthy.

**Losing weight is a healing journey.**

In that moment, it dawned on me that, '*losing weight is a healing journey.*' It seemed so simple. Why hadn't anyone shared this with me before?

Inspired by my initial results I continued to pursue my natural health and healing goals. Within 12 months, a medical report confirmed what I already knew; I was in a state of excellent health, with normal blood sugar levels and healthy functioning organs including my liver, kidneys, thyroid and adrenal glands.

A second medical report a few years later pronounced me 100% asthma free. That was a special day in my life!

My weight continued to fall off. I ended up losing over 60 pounds of excess body weight and have successfully kept it off for over 12 years now. I achieved all of these long-lasting results with no medications, drugs, deprivation, harmful side effects, counting calories, weighing food, portion control or surgery.

**Finding food freedom.**

After embracing the path of health and wellness in my own life, today I feel more vibrant, alive and younger than ever before. My healing journey forced me out of my comfort zone and into the unknown. I now allow my life to unfold effortlessly around me. Every day, I feel filled with gratitude for the many gifts that have shown up in my life.

Being sick, fat and tired was one of the biggest challenges of my life. I now know that it was my opportunity to learn and grow so I could create and experience the life that I truly desired.

I feel so blessed today to be able to share my story with women from all over the world, through my yoga retreats, writing, teaching, coaching and healing work.

**You have the power to lose weight naturally.**

When you focus upon healing your body, mind and emotions you will lose weight naturally and permanently.

Over the course of this book I will share the same health and healing principles that I personally applied to bring my life back into balance. These healing principles enabled me to lose weight naturally, feel good about myself and start enjoying my life again.

If you apply these same principles in your own life, I know that you too can do the same.

# The problem with dieting.

*"The definition of insanity is doing the same thing over and over and expecting different results."*

*~ Albert Einstein*

It is widely accepted that '95% of all diets fail', resulting in long term weight gain and lowered self esteem. And yet, despite these appalling statistics, 4 out of every 10 women in the United Kingdom are permanently on some form of diet.

Let's face it; our collective addiction to dieting really is a dark comedy bordering on the edge of the absurd. Think of it this way. If you had a class full of enthusiastic students and 95% of them routinely failed their exams, would you say that the problem resided with the students or with the teaching methodology?

The dieting mentality would suggest that the students are at fault and should be the ones to blame. But when we allow ourselves to take a closer look, perhaps it is the teaching methodology that has been failing the students?

### Dieting doesn't address the real problem.

The reason why the dieting approach has such a high failure rate is because it focuses upon all the wrong issues. No amount of calorie counting and mindless exercise can resolve the inner issues relating to a woman's body image, self esteem, intimate relationships or family life.

Many women I have spoken to who struggle with their weight, can reel off all the different diets that they have tried. For the most part, these diets fall into some permutation of the popular dieting model of 'eat less, exercise more'. This model is so well known and accepted that if you ask most people who haven't had a weight problem why people are overweight, they will often say it is because they either 'eat too much' or they 'don't exercise enough'.

And yet, many women who diet regularly are quick to point out that they don't eat significantly more food than skinny women. Very often they also have a regular exercise program as well. But still they struggle to shift those unwanted pounds to experience the natural and permanent weight loss they desire.

Now while I certainly agree that diet and exercise have an important role to play in the weight loss journey, what I have discovered is that if you focus on them (to the exclusion of the other important aspects of weight loss and healing) you will almost certainly end up more overweight than when you began.

On my own weight loss journey, the 'eat less and exercise more', although making logical sense, was never able to yield the long term results that I was desperately searching for. And I know this holds true for many women. Whenever I lost weight by trying to control my diet and exercise, whilst ignoring the inner aspects of my being, regardless of any short term results that would transpire, life would inevitably get in the way.

Boredom, stress, emotional upset or just plain hunger would kick in and I would feel compelled to break my diet and exercise routine. This would always result in me binging on my favourite comfort foods and regaining any weight that I had just lost.

**Dieting is a cycle of self abuse.**

Dieting is a physically, mentally and emotionally abusive approach to losing weight. The 'dieting cycle' is a highly sophisticated one that very few women manage to break out of. It has been purposefully engineered by companies that have a vested interest in keeping you stuck, confused and overweight.

Breaking free of this mentality is like leaving an abusive job or relationship. When you leave it behind you, you will wonder why you didn't do it sooner.

You can tell the quality of any relationship simply by the way that it makes you feel about yourself. For most women this relationship to dieting is a loathsome one.

My own dieting trigger used to get activated whenever I reached the last notch on my belt or when I could no longer bear to look at myself in the mirror. My self imposed diet would commence in earnest. I remember relentlessly trying to follow low calorie eating plans that were probably more aptly described as 'starvation plans'.

Despite my best intentions, I would soon be overcome with uncontrollable urges to ditch my diet and binge on the closest chocolate bar I could get my hands on. All changes I made to the way that I ate were temporary. Over time this pattern wreaked havoc upon my self esteem and confidence, as well as my waist line.

Dieting put an increasing strain on my already tenuous relationship with food and my body. These once dear friends had somehow become my enemies.

The yo-yo dieting cycle was an emotional roller coaster for me. It wrapped me up in an unfolding sequence of deprivation, desire, frustration, embarrassment, guilt, anger and ultimately shame.

The one thing that I couldn't see at the time was that dieting was a regime that I had ultimately inflicted upon myself.

**Dieting makes you fat.**

For women wanting to lose weight, they are often told that their only option is to 'go on a diet'. But dieting typically results in women actually gaining weight, creating the opposite effect of what they originally wanted. How it this even possible?

This happens due to the restrictive nature of dieting. When you deprive your body of adequate nutrition it becomes vulnerable to variable energy, sickness and disease.

When losing weight, it is important to eat food regularly to maintain a healthy metabolism. The dieting approach can actually result in interfering and negatively affecting your body's natural cycles.

When you diet, you are effectively starving your body of nutrition. With reduced nutrients, food and energy intake, your instinctive survival program is kick started. Your body is led to believe that it must survive on minimal food. The sophistication of your body's inner intelligence is notched up a gear. Your body will start to retain water and store fat, to ensure that you have adequate nutrients in case your survival is threatened.

It is easy to prevent this extreme form of survival program from being activated. Simply avoid harmful dieting and weight loss approaches that focus exclusively on reducing calories and restricting your food intake.

You want your body to function optimally in a way that is in flow with your own natural rhythms and cycles. When you place your body in the wrong environment, expose it to the wrong foods, your weight and your health will certainly be compromised. Too much stress or stimulants, coupled with not enough sleep will overwork your body's immune system and negatively impact your health.

As you are about to learn, you can lose weight naturally by healing your body with the right nutrients, fluids, gentle movement and appropriate rest. Your body and health can rebalance very quickly when you provide it with these types of natural healing tools.

When your body is adequately nourished it is able to function normally and will begin the process of self healing.

**A flawed model in need of revolution.**

The dieting approach is a deeply flawed model in need of revolution. The important thing to realise at this stage, is that there is an alternative.

'Ditching your dieting mentality' frees you from the feelings of deprivation, desire and guilt, without subjecting yourself to the abuse that is so commonly associated with dieting. Doing this is a very conscious process and a deep act of self love. It will enable you to create a healthy relationship with food, your body and yourself.

When you 'ditch your dieting mentality', you open the doorway to internal peace, freedom and kindness. You deserve to live a life free from self punishment and attack. It is a gift that only you can give yourself.

Taking a healing approach to losing weight is the break-through that you have been searching for. I lost over 60 pounds by 'ditching my dieting mentality' and in the process I radically transformed my own life. I know that if you follow the healing approach to losing weight that is contained within this book, that you can naturally and permanently lose weight too.

# A healing approach to losing weight.

*"You did what you knew how to do, and when you knew better, you did better."*

*~ Maya Angelou*

*'Losing Weight is a Healing Journey'* is an invitation to heal yourself from the inside out. It is a total paradigm shift away from the collective hypnosis that women have been subjected to through the traditional model of dieting. The weight loss journey is one that allows you to discover your true potential by gently releasing the past and taking a healing approach to your life.

The majority of dieting approaches would have you believe that you are just a physical body, but the reality is that you are so much more than this. Beyond your physical self are the non-physical aspects of your nature including your thoughts, beliefs and emotions. These aspects hold the key to why you gained weight in the first place and also what you can do to lose it.

This book is structured around the three key phases of the weight loss healing journey. These are:

Phase 1: Heal your body.

Phase 2: Heal your mind.

Phase 3: Heal your emotions.

I have written this book in a way that mirrors my own personal experience. On my own journey I made the decision to turn my focus away from dieting, deprivation and portion control. Instead I turned my attention towards my health, healing and wellness and this is what made all the difference.

Throughout this book I share the ideas, tools and techniques that helped me to bring my life and body back into balance whilst losing weight naturally in the process.

**Your 'Inner' and 'Outer' worlds.**

I want you to take a moment to imagine an iceberg. Can you picture those big blocks of ice jutting straight out of the ocean?

The iceberg that we see sitting on the surface of the ocean is really only the 'tip' of the iceberg. What most people don't realise is that about 80% of the iceberg itself is submerged and hidden deep beneath the sea.

And so it is with weight loss. The dieting approach focuses upon the visible aspects of weight loss or what I call the 'Outer World' whilst disregarding the 'Inner World'.

The Outer World of weight loss is made up of food, exercise and your physical body. Although these aspects are important, they only ever reveal a small part of the story.

What is sitting beneath the surface and unaddressed by most dieting approaches is the Inner World. The Inner World of weight loss includes your thoughts, beliefs and emotions. It is here, in your Inner World that you will find the real secret to losing weight naturally and keeping it off for good.

When you take a healing approach to losing weight, you bring unity and balance to both your Inner and Outer worlds.


**Your weight loss healing journey.**

When you change your focus from dieting to healing, your life will change forever. You will start to uncover the answers that have seemingly eluded you. Of course you will be tested along the way but once you become aware of this you can rise above any challenge you encounter on your path.

Your weight loss healing journey will give you the opportunity to learn and discover many new things about yourself. You will also strengthen who you are and increase your levels of self-awareness.

When you apply the ideas contained within *'Losing Weight is a Healing Journey'* not only will you lose weight naturally but your life will just work better. By taking a healing approach to weight loss you can set yourself free; physically, mentally and emotionally.

**The Dieting Approach vs. The Healing Approach.**

The following chart gives you a summary of the healing approach to weight loss compared to the dieting approach.

| The Dieting Approach to Weight Loss | The Healing Approach to Weight Loss |
|---|---|
| ✗ Focus on quick fixes | ✓ Focus on permanent results |
| ✗ Rigid, dogmatic and prescriptive | ✓ Flexible, intuitive and non prescriptive |
| ✗ Follow the dieting 'experts' | ✓ Become your own authority |
| ✗ Formulaic approach | ✓ Unique to each person |
| ✗ Dishonours the body's wisdom | ✓ Honours the body's wisdom |
| ✗ Something is wrong with the body | ✓ The body always gives accurate feedback |
| ✗ Disempowers the individual | ✓ Empowers the individual |
| ✗ Target fat and problem areas | ✓ Support holistic healing |
| ✗ Ignores real reasons for weight gain | ✓ Opportunity to develop self awareness |
| ✗ A masculine approach | ✓ A feminine approach |

# PHASE 1:

# Heal Your Body

# Chapter One – Food

*"To eat is a necessity; to eat intelligently is an art."*

*~ La Rochefoucauld*

| The Dieting Approach to Weight Loss | The Healing Approach to Weight Loss |
|---|---|
| ✗ Food is the problem | ✓ Food is an important part of the solution |
| ✗ Eat low calorie foods | ✓ Eat real foods that nourish your body |
| ✗ Focus on food restriction | ✓ Focus on food freedom |
| ✗ Food makes you fat | ✓ Food heals your body |
| ✗ A short term, crash approach | ✓ A long term, sustainable approach |
| ✗ Portion control and restriction | ✓ Eat an abundance of natural foods |

## Rule 1: Eat consciously.

*"Did you ever stop to taste a carrot? Not just eat it, but taste it? You can't taste the beauty and energy of the earth in a Twinkie."*

*~ Astrid Alauda*

True and deep healing happens in the presence of awareness. The act of bringing conscious awareness to the foods you eat, as well as your eating patterns, will help you to connect to your body's needs and rhythms.

When I started out on my weight loss healing journey, one of the first things that my naturopath did was draw my attention to the power of food to either harm or heal my body.

She asked me to start becoming more conscious of the foods that I was eating and the physical, mental and emotional affects that they were having upon me.

**So what does eating consciously mean?**

Eating consciously is about being mindful of the foods that you eat and making the connection to how food affects you. It is about choosing to eat in a way that feels empowering and uplifting for you. Conscious eating is a way to tune into your own body so that you can make food choices that support your long term health and wellness.

As you become more conscious of your food choices and eating patterns, you will start to build a much healthier relationship with food. You will start to appreciate the food that you eat more whilst also savouring all the many different tastes, textures and flavours of food.

Recently I facilitated a week long 'Yoga and Detox' program at a retreat centre in Urbino, Italy. One of the practices for the week was to learn how to eat more consciously. To achieve this, we dedicated an entire lunch to eating in silence.

Afterwards, it was fascinating to hear what people had to share about the experience, particularly from those people who were slightly apprehensive about the experiment. Many people shared that they discovered profound things about themselves. Some of the insightful comments participants offered to the group included: *'I ate less'*, *'I felt like I was really able to savour the taste of my food'*, *'My food tasted sweeter'*, *'I really noticed when I was beginning to feel full'* and *'I was able to eat with the desires of my stomach instead of my eyes!'*

Other things you can do to start eating more consciously include:

- Give thanks and appreciation for your food.
- Chew your food properly.
- Slow down to taste your food.
- Use cutlery when eating your meals.
- Stop eating when you are full.

**What is unconscious eating?**

When you eat unconsciously, there is a natural disassociation between the food you consume and how it affects your health, energy levels and waistline. This style of eating can also be described as 'mindless eating' and can easily occur when you are feeling tired, stressed, anxious or distracted. When you eat unconsciously you can lose focus upon 'what' as well as 'how much' food you are eating.

Have you ever had the experience of eating something without having any memory of eating it? Does food somehow mysteriously vanish in your presence? Can you eat a whole block of chocolate without even noticing? These are all tell-tale signs of unconscious eating patterns.

Unconscious food consumption patterns can include eating while:

- Sitting in front of the television.
- Working on the computer.
- Talking on the phone.
- Feeling stressed or distracted.
- Driving your car.

Breaking these patterns of unconscious eating can transform the way you live forever. Creating simple rules for yourself like not eating in front of the television or sitting at your desk can help tremendously.

At the height of my weight problems I found myself stuck in a chronic pattern of unconscious eating. Due to my busy schedule and tendency to cram too much into my day, I would habitually be forced to override my body's natural desire for proper nutrition by skipping meals. To compensate for this, I would unconsciously eat food on the run, during meetings or while I was working.

## Becoming conscious of when you eat.

An important aspect of becoming more conscious of the food you eat is paying attention to the times that you eat. I find that what works best for me is to have a big breakfast, morning snacks, a hearty lunch, afternoon snacks and a small dinner early in the evening.

Try to eat your evening dinner, at least 3 hours before you go to bed. As a regular practice, don't eat late at night and certainly don't make eating late at night a regular habit. When you go to bed on a full stomach your body focuses on digesting food rather than healing and rejuvenation. When you wake up, have a big breakfast early in the morning. As a result you may find that you experience much better quality sleep and as a result need less of it.

Your body will love you for going to bed on an empty stomach. This allows your body to focus upon cleansing and healing, rather than digestion.

## Broader concerns of food issues.

As you become more conscious of your own eating habits, you may feel moved to explore wider issues around the way we produce food in our modern world.

Things you may begin to think about and question include:

- Who grew my food?
- How was it grown?
- What country does my food come from?
- How old is my food by the time it reaches me?
- Were any chemicals used in the production of my food?

**Before and after.**

One of the most common questions I get from women who are curious about my weight loss transformation is about what I used to eat versus what I eat now. Or in other words, what kind of foods I ate when I was eating unconsciously versus the foods that I consciously started to eat to bring my body back into balance.

Here is a simple chart that summarises the foods that I would typically eat 'before' and 'whilst' I lost weight.

| Katrina's typical food day comparison. | | |
|---|---|---|
| | **Before losing weight.** | **Whilst I lost weight.** |
| **Breakfast** | *Time: 10am*<br>Coffee<br>Muffin or<br>Croissant or<br>Danish pastry or<br>White bread roll | *Time: 8am*<br>Lemon water<br>Coffee substitute<br>Fruit salad or<br>Porridge with soy milk or<br>Bircher muesli or<br>Poached eggs on spinach or<br>Scrambled eggs on toast |
| **Morning snack** | *Time: 12pm*<br>Low fat muesli bar or<br>Protein bar | *Time: 10am*<br>Vegetables and humus or<br>Vegetables and dip or<br>Green smoothie |
| **Lunch** | *Time: 3pm*<br>Pastry and coffee or<br>Low fat 'diet' yogurt or<br>Bagel with cream cheese | *Time: 12pm*<br>Fish and green salad or<br>Chicken and vegetables or<br>Salmon sushi with salad |

| | | |
|---|---|---|
| **Afternoon snack** | *Time: 6pm*<br>Chocolate biscuit & tea or<br>Chocolate bar or<br>Protein bar or<br>A glass of wine and nibbles | *Time: 3pm*<br>Miso soup or<br>Dried fruit or<br>Dark chocolate or<br>Seasoned pumpkin seeds |
| **Dinner** | *Time: 9pm*<br>Hot chips or<br>Vegetarian kebab or<br>Indian take-away | *Time: 6pm*<br>Salad with tofu / chicken stir fry or<br>Salad with fish curry and brown rice or<br>Vegetable soup |
| **After Dinner** | *Time: 11pm*<br>Hot chocolate and biscuits | No food 3 hours before bed. |
| **Water consumed** | 1 - 2 glasses of water per day | 6 - 8 glasses of water per day |

# Exercise: Keep a food diary.

1. Use the 'Your weekly food diary' worksheet (see example overleaf) to keep track of the foods that you consume over the course of a week.

2. What interesting things did you discover about your eating patterns and habits through this process?

.................................................................................

| Your weekly food diary. | | | | | | | |
|---|---|---|---|---|---|---|---|
| | Mon | Tues | Wed | Thu | Fri | Sat | Sun |
| **Breakfast** | | | | | | | |
| **Morning snack** | | | | | | | |
| **Lunch** | | | | | | | |
| **Afternoon snack** | | | | | | | |
| **Dinner** | | | | | | | |
| **Evening snack** | | | | | | | |

# Rule 2: Eat real foods.

*"If you can't say it, don't eat it."*

*~ Michael Pollan*

If you want to lose weight naturally it is essential that you eat foods that your body recognises as food. Permanent weight loss is more about focusing upon 'what kinds' of food you eat rather than 'how much' you eat.

Your body needs real foods to create long term health and vitality. The old adage holds true, 'you are what you eat.' The food you put in your mouth really does affect you.

The radical industrialisation of the food chain, which has occurred over the past 50 years, has transformed a largely natural, organic and local food production cycle into an artificially created, mechanised, global one.

There has been a massive departure away from the connection that our ancestors had with the land, food production and preparation. With the constraints of modern day living, most people today have no idea how their food is produced or about the chain of events that occur prior to their food appearing before them.

The Academy Award nominated documentary called *'Food Inc: How industrial food is making us sicker, fatter and poorer - and what you can do about it'*, reveals that our food production methods have changed more in the last 50 years, than they have done in the preceding 10,000 years. During this same time period, we have witnessed an alarming increase in chronic health conditions such as cancer, diabetes, heart disease and obesity.

Today, food production has become a matter of profits and big business. This bottom line focus has come at the expense of your health, well being and your waistline.

In 2007, the UK Government-commissioned Foresight report predicted that, 'if no action was taken, 60% of men, 50% of women and 25% of children would be obese by 2050.'

The dieting industry has hypnotised us into focusing our full attention upon calorie counting and portion control. They have achieved this whilst getting us to ignore the things that really matter: nutrient levels of food, natural food production methods and preparing food with love.

## Overcoming confusion around food.

From personal experience I know how confusing and overwhelming the area of food can be. It is quite amazing that something so simple has become so hard to understand.

It is no wonder when you realise that today, there are approximately 20,000 - 40,000 food items in an average British supermarket, giving us more food choices than ever before.

People in the US find themselves in a similar predicament. Marion Nestle author of the *'The soft sell: how the food industry shapes our diets'* in 2002, says "The average number of products carried by a typical US supermarket has more than tripled since 1980, from 15,000 to 50,000.

In 1998 alone, manufacturers introduced more than 11,000 new foods. More than two-thirds of them were condiments, candy and snacks, baked goods, soft drinks, cheese products and ice cream novelties."

This culture of seemingly endless food choices has resulted in mass confusion and this has created an environment where so many women routinely give away their power.

Knowing what to eat is perhaps the most confusing thing that women have to deal with on the path to losing weight. I know I found it confusing. Like many women, I had been faithfully following the dieting approach to losing weight with pretty lack-lustre results.

When I was rebuilding my health, I realised that I had to change my whole approach to food.

What I needed was a practical philosophy that was easy to understand and follow that would help me to make better food choices.

To achieve this, I started to classify food into 3 basic categories: *'real foods', 'lightly processed foods'* and *'fake foods'.*

I then applied the following guideline to increase my consumption of real foods.

(a) Eat 80% real foods.
(b) Eat 20% lightly processed foods.
(c) Substitute fake foods.

The 'eat 80% real foods' is a simple guideline to assist you to make healthy food choices for yourself. It is the same one that I applied to radically transform my health and permanently lose 60 pounds in the process.

The key element to keep in mind with these guidelines is the fact that they are there to help you to focus your attention upon the thing that is most important. Stephen Covey author of '*The 7 habits of highly effective people*' said it best when he wrote: "the main thing is, to keep the main thing, the main thing". The main thing that I want you to take from this section is simply 'eat more real foods'.

Use this as a guideline for sustainable and healthy living. Just know that for most women this change is not likely to occur overnight. If you still chose to occasionally eat 'fake foods' or a higher percentage of 'lightly processed foods' just notice how it makes you feel afterwards.

When I started to apply these guidelines in my own life, I noticed that my body and energy levels improved. This motivated me to want to eat more real food. I learnt that not only does my body feel more energised but I actually preferred the taste of real and lightly processed foods to that of highly manufactured fake foods.

We will explore these three food guidelines in more detail below.

## 1. Eat 80% real foods.

Eating real foods means eating whole natural foods that haven't been tampered with, just as nature intended. Real foods nourish the body and support its ability to detoxify and self heal.

Real foods grow naturally on trees, in vegetable gardens, paddocks, lakes, rivers or in the ocean. They are rich in nutrients absorbed from the soil, sunshine, water and fresh air.

They are the types of foods that your grandparents used to eat before the mass scale corporatisation and industrialisation of food production. They are the foods that your body recognises and can be most readily digested.

Allow your food intake to come from 80% real foods. This may appear like quite a leap when you are starting out. Just know that the consumption of real foods is the building blocks for creating true health and vitality.

One thing I personally did to make this target more achievable was to spend more time cooking for myself at home, instead of buying food on the run.

Examples of real foods include:

- Fresh fruit.
- Fresh leafy greens, vegetables and seaweeds.
- Whole grains such as brown rice, millet, polenta and quinoa.
- Legumes, beans, pulses, lentils, nuts and seeds.
- Natural flavourings such as sea salt and honey.
- Organic red meat, chicken, fish and eggs.

## 2. Eat 20% lightly processed foods.

Lightly processed foods are foods made from real ingredients, which have been naturally processed and packaged within the food chain before you eat them.

These foods do not contain harmful chemicals, such as artificial flavourings, colourings, additives and preservatives. When you read the ingredients listed on the packaging you recognise them and can easily pronounce them.

Lightly processed foods are frequently produced by health conscious companies that have an innate awareness of the problems that are associated with artificially processed foods. They produce their food using healthy food preparation methods and their ingredients are derived from real foods.

Allow 20% of your food intake to come from lightly processed foods. This one rule will give you the flexibility you need to design a long term and nourishing way of eating that will help you to naturally lose weight for good.

Examples of lightly processed foods include:

- Naturally baked whole grain breads and pastas.
- Jars of olives, peppers, sundried tomatoes and artichokes.
- Extra virgin olive oil and extra virgin coconut oil.

- Tins of lentils, beans and chickpeas.
- Hummus, tahini and tamari.
- Organic teas and coffees.
- Organic dairy and cheeses.
- Soya, almond and rice milk.
- Organic chocolate.
- Dried fruits.

## 3. Avoid fake foods.

Most people are familiar with the term 'junk food'. The 'fake food' definition broadens the 'junk food' definition to include many of the pre-packaged snacks, processed meals and 'diet foods' that exist on the market today.

'Fake foods' are foods that contain ingredients that have been artificially created or chemically altered, through the use of artificial additives, preservatives, colourings, flavourings, stabilisers, thickeners, emulsifiers, sweeteners, trans-fatty acids, refined fats, high corn fructose syrup (HCFS), glucose-fructose syrup and e-numbers. They include all foods that have been heavily processed and are removed from their natural state.

Food manufacturers engineer fake foods to maximise shelf life, reduce costs and to create addiction. This is all done ultimately to enhance profit. Despite any marketing claims to the contrary, these foods have not been created with the intention of generating health or wellbeing for you or your family.

It is important to realise that these 'fake foods' are not 'real foods' as they are toxic and harmful to your long term health. They are also a major contributing factor in weight gain.

A good way to avoid fake foods is to avoid processed foods that contain ingredients that you can't pronounce.

This one guideline can pretty much help you to take a big leap forward to increasing your intake of real foods.

As an alternative, simply look for a similar product made from natural ingredients.

Examples of fake foods that I substituted included:

- Ready-made meals and diet foods made with artificial ingredients.
- White bread and baked goods made with bleached flour.
- Soft drinks made with sugar or artificial sweeteners.
- Snack foods seasoned with iodised table salt.
- Deep fried foods and fast foods, high in trans-fats.
- Non-organic meat and dairy foods.

## Fake foods make you fat.

Regularly eating fake foods, regardless of how many calories they contain or how low they are in fat or sugar, is a recipe for poor health and weight gain.

Fake foods harm the natural functioning of your body particularly your body's digestive system. They are extremely difficult for your body to break down and eliminate. The main reason being that your body doesn't recognise them as food.

In the Academy award nominated documentary called 'Super Size Me', filmmaker Morgan Spurlock undertakes a 30-day body experiment of exclusively eating 3 meals of McDonald's per day. If you haven't had a chance to see this movie, I highly recommend that you watch it.

By the end of the film he had gained 25 pounds (11 kg), suffered liver dysfunction and depression (he was above-average health and fitness when he started the film). After the experiment was complete, it took Spurlock fourteen months to return back to his normal weight of 185 pounds (84 kg).

## Making better food decisions.

When was the last time that you saw an animal in its natural habitat consulting a diet book in order to work out what to eat? It doesn't happen because instinctually animals know exactly what to eat. If a wild animal comes across something that it doesn't recognise as food it won't eat it.

This also holds true for domesticated animals too. Recent experiments have shown that when cows are given the choice of either an organic feed or a genetically modified (GMO) feed, they will instinctively choose the natural, organic one.

The good news is that you have the same instincts around food. Your body can tell the difference between what is good for you and what isn't. These natural food instincts however have been submerged beneath a sea of bogus scientific food research, false advertising and marketing hype.

The majority of what you see promoted through 'food industry' marketing campaigns are fake foods, with well-known, popular brand names. I mean when was the last TV marketing campaign developed to promote the importance of eating broccoli?

It is a scary fact that more money is often spent on advertising and marketing fake food than is spent on producing it. These fake 'food marketing' messages are often intentionally misleading by omitting the most important and basic facts about the food and how it was produced.

Spurious marketing claims such as 'fat free', 'cholesterol free', 'no added sugar', 'added vitamins and minerals' or 'zero calories' lead many women to mistakenly believe that they are eating something healthy. For the most part this is just not the case. If the food you are about to eat is a fake food, just know that it is doing your body harm and placing your long term health and weight loss plans at risk.

The one thing you can be reassured of is that your body always knows the truth.


**Real foods are healing foods.**


Now is the time to start making better food decisions for yourself. To make better food choices you need to become aware of whether something is a 'real food', 'lightly processed food' or a 'fake food'.

To become more mindful of what is contained within the food you eat, begin to read the ingredients on food packaging. This will help you to navigate marketing claims, avoid fake foods and choose real foods instead. Eating real foods are the building blocks that are required to create a healthy and trim body. Simply by eating real food, your body will begin to detoxify and naturally heal, as well as shed excess weight.

When you eat more real foods, such as vegetables (especially green leafy vegetables), fruit, whole grains, beans and legumes you will also lose weight naturally and permanently. Being prepared and having real food close at hand will make eating it much easier for you.

As a society, we have become disassociated from the foods that we eat. Fewer people grow their own food or prepare their meals from scratch. Even sitting down to enjoy a family meal at the table is fast becoming a thing of the past.

Eating at least 80% real foods combined with 20% lightly processed foods, gives you a sustainable eating plan that you can follow for life. Eating in this way will put you on the path to healing your weight problems and creating true health from within.

When you eat real whole foods, not only will your body love you forever, you will create a vibrant, healthy and happy body. Your body is your temple. It is your home. Treat it well and it will treat you well.

# Exercise: Where are you now?

1. In the chart below, take a moment to estimate what is the breakdown of your food consumption between the following 3 food categories:

|  | Real foods | Lightly processed foods | Fake foods |
|---|---|---|---|
| **Target** | 80% | 20% | Avoid |
| **Current** |  |  |  |

The next chart shows the shopping list that I use to ensure that I always have an abundance of real foods in my kitchen cupboards at all times.

# Katrina's 'Real Food' shopping list:

**Seasonal greens**

- Rocket, sprouts, kale, lettuce, spinach, mustard greens, collards, celery, broccoli, cabbage, cucumbers, zucchini/courgettes, avocado.

**Fresh vegetables**

- Garlic, ginger, carrots, onions, peppers, pumpkin, sweet potato, beetroot, leeks, aubergines and fresh herbs.

**Protein sources (Organic)**

- Tofu, free-range eggs, Sun warrior vegetarian protein powder.

**Fresh and dried fruit**

- Lemons, grapefruit, limes, kiwifruit, berries, bananas, apples, watermelon, pineapple, tomatoes, melons, mangos.
- Dried apricots (preservative free), raisins, figs, prunes, dates.

**Flavourings and seasonings**

- Hummus, pesto, tahini, curry paste, miso, sundried tomatoes.
- Apple cider vinegar, tamari, sea salt, coconut water, nut butter, cocoa, carob, vanilla essence.

**Whole grains and legumes**

- Spelt, brown rice, lentils, couscous, buckwheat or rice noodles, oats, quinoa, millet, polenta, split peas, kelp noodles, chickpeas.

**Oils, seeds and nuts**

- Extra virgin olive oil, extra virgin coconut oil, organic butter.
- Sunflower seeds, sesame seeds, chia seeds, pumpkin seeds, flax seed, brazil nuts, pine nuts, almonds, walnuts, pecans, cashew nuts.

**Super foods and sweeteners.**

- Chlorella and spirulina tablets/powder, seaweed.
- Honey, stevia, maple syrup, coconut nectar, dark chocolate.

# Rule 3: Substitution not deprivation.

*"The commonest form of malnutrition in the western world is obesity."*

*~ Mervyn Deitel*

Once you are able to classify your possible food choices into either *'real foods'*, *'lightly processed foods'* and *'fake foods'*, your focus then shifts to upgrading your food choices wherever possible.

The important thing to grasp here is that all food is not created equal. How your food has been cooked along with how it has been prepared makes all the difference. For example a hamburger could be healing or harmful for your body, depending on how it has been made and the ingredients it has been made with.

The Mayor of New York, Michael Bloomberg, recently remarked, *"Nobody wants to take away your French fries or hamburgers – I love these things too, but if you can make them from ingredients that are less damaging to your health we should do that."*

Unfortunately, we live in a world today where a high percentage of food is heavily processed. Much of this food is cheap and frequently discounted when bought in bulk.

On a positive note, things are starting to change. Healthier food options are beginning to emerge. For example, many petrol stations in the UK are being transformed with the addition of mini-supermarkets which stock a variety of different healthy food options for consumers.

**From deprivation to food freedom.**

One of the main reasons why the dieting model doesn't work is because it is based upon restriction, deprivation and control.

Whenever you remove something from your diet, it is important that you replace or substitute it with a healthier and more nourishing option. If you just remove the food item without replacing it with something else, you will more than likely experience cravings for it or withdrawal symptoms from it. In some cases it may even work to deepen the desire for the thing that you stopped eating. In extreme cases, this type of behaviour can set up a cycle of addiction that can be much harder to break out of.

By substituting the fake foods that I had been eating for nutritious foods, I found that I could free myself from the torture of counting calories, weighing food or measuring portions. By eating healthy servings of nutritious food, I no longer felt as if I was missing out. If my body was hungry, I knew that I had plenty of real food options to choose from.

I approached substitution with a sense of curiosity and light-heartedness. In doing so, I was able to break free of the feelings of deprivation that I had suffered from when I was dieting. Using the approach of substitution, I changed my relationship with myself and I began to feel powerful around food.

Many of my weight loss break-through clients share this experience. Below is an email that I received from Alani:

*"Yesterday I went shopping after work... while shopping I was looking at the foods I used to buy (so called fat free stuff etc) and started thinking about my new approach to food - eating whole and real foods... I felt so happy... I felt brightened up. I felt excited to get home and try something. Like... I found some South African pears and I chomped it up like it was the best thing I ever ate... I had that free feeling when unpacking the groceries..."*

As Alani opened her mind to substitution and not deprivation she was able to see a whole range of food choices that she previously hadn't noticed.

**Changing your relationship to food.**

One of the best ways I found to wean myself off high processed foods and drinks is to research them. In many cases, when you learn how these foods are produced you will not want to eat them. Knowledge is power. For example when I learnt about what happened to caged hens I realised that I could only buy free-range, organic eggs.

Substitution will allow you to create a great relationship with food so that you can enjoy eating again. You know that you are not only satisfying your taste buds, but you are also building the cells of a wonderful new body.

There are a huge variety of healing foods that are available that taste delicious. When I teach my 'Yoga and Detox' retreats, I get my students to focus upon eating real food. One of the things that participants comment upon is how amazing they feel from eating real wholesome foods. Many are surprised about how much real food they could eat and still lose weight!

On my own weight loss journey, once I started to look for healing foods, I was amazed at all the number of delicious foods that I found. I came to really enjoy the process of discovering real and lightly processed food in health food shops, farmer's markets and delicatessens. In the health section of my local supermarket I also found many interesting foods that I had never seen before, along with new healthy recipes to try.

**Focus on what you can eat.**

The key to making this transition work for you is by focusing your attention on the abundance of amazing foods you 'can eat'. When you use the power of substitution it means that you get to experience feeling really good about yourself while you are eating as well as after you finish eating. You will feel light and energized with no bloating, gas, nausea, water retention or fatigue.

Simply changing your focus from 'cannot eat' to 'can eat', will make a significant difference to your health and state of mind. As a result, you will notice changes in your energy levels, waist line and the bathroom scales too.

Your body will certainly notice a difference. It can easily digest and absorb the nutrients that can be found in whole foods. Substituting fake foods for foods made with real ingredients that your body recognises, will have the immediate effect of natural, healthy and permanent weight loss.

Below is a chart that you can use to help you substitute harmful, fake foods out of your life and instead replace them with 'real foods' or 'lightly processed foods'.

# Fake food substitutions.

Listed below are some common fake foods (highly processed foods), which I recommend that you substitute out of your life and replace them with real or lightly processed foods instead.

| Fake Foods | Real or Lightly Processed Foods |
|---|---|
| Muffins, cakes or biscuits | • Wheat, gluten and sugar free options<br>• Explore raw desserts and sweets |
| White Bread | • Brown or rye bread<br>• Gluten free breads with spelt or rice flour<br>• Organic, whole grain baked goods |
| Crisps / chips | • Baked, not fried chips<br>• Pumpkin seeds cooked in tamari (soy sauce)<br>• Home-made potato wedges<br>• Baked or roasted vegetable chips |
| Ice cream | • Dairy free soy, rice or coconut ice-cream<br>• Organic ice-cream<br>• Frozen sorbet |
| Cheese | • Sheep or goats cheese<br>• Raw cheese<br>• Seed and nut cheese |
| Chocolate | • Organic chocolate<br>• Dark chocolate (70% cocoa)<br>• Raw chocolate<br>• Carob |

| | |
|---|---|
| Cooked breakfasts | • Porridge<br>• Scrambled or poached eggs on spinach<br>• Roasted tomatoes, grilled mushrooms, avocado and fresh herbs with goat's cheese |
| Creamy sauces | • Olive oil, garlic, lemon juice and fresh herbs<br>• Tomato herb sauce<br>• Tomato, chilli and basil sauce |
| Pizza | • Top a heated thin pizza base with generous amounts of rocket, lettuce, pesto, sundried or fresh tomatoes and basil |
| Coffee | • Drink less: order a small or medium sized cup<br>• Drink high quality, organic coffee<br>• Coffee substitute: teeccino, caro<br>• Dandelion coffee, immune boosting Reishi mushroom coffee, herbal tea |
| Alcohol | • Drink less: order a small glass of wine<br>• Drink high quality, organic alcohol<br>• Non-alcoholic wine or cocktails. One of my favourites drinks is soda water, fresh mint, lime & lemon |
| Soft drinks | • Drink still or sparkling water<br>• Fresh water with lemon, mint and fruit (such as oranges, cucumber, and pineapple)<br>• Make healthy soft drinks at home (lemon, lime, honey and ginger)<br>• Fresh vegetable juices |

**Reading ingredient lists.**

By law, food manufacturers must list what ingredients they add to their products to make them. In theory, that should make it easy to know which foods you want to buy. But often these companies use very sneaky methods to conceal the ingredients that they use.

Ingredients are always listed in descending order of product by weight. So when you read an ingredient list, you know that the first ingredient listed is what the product is mostly made from.

Do not look at the products advertising claims on the package. Many people are easily misled by the terminology that food companies use.

For example, be careful to make sure you are buying whole wheat bread. Check that the ingredient list states that the flour is 100% whole wheat. Many companies use words such as 'wheat flour', 'unbleached wheat flour', 'multigrain', 'enriched or stone ground wheat flour' instead of saying 'refined white flour'.

Another thing to watch out for when you read food ingredient lists is a sweetener called high corn fructose syrup (in the UK it is called glucose-fructose syrup). It is commonly used in processed foods. It is a highly refined sweetener made from corn with many studies linking it to the rise in obesity and weight gain statistics, along with chronic health conditions. Most fake foods are high in this ingredient.

Once you start paying attention to the ingredients contained in your foods, you will able to find brands and food items that you can trust.

Healthy food companies, as well as using real foods in their products, prepare their food using natural preparation methods where possible. They focus on operating ethically, treating their food, customers and employees with care and love. Spend your money wisely by buying food that helps to make the world a healthier place to live.

To give you an example of 'Substitution not Elimination' in action, here is a food comparison chart. It shows how certain foods can be made using either real foods, lightly processed foods or fake foods, depending upon the ingredients used to produce them.

| Food Comparison Chart. | | | |
|---|---|---|---|
| **Food** | **Real Food** | **Lightly Processed** | **Fake Food** |
| **BBQ sauce** | *Homemade BBQ sauce.* Tomatoes, onion, molasses, vinegar, red pepper flakes, sugar, sea salt, garlic, mustard, olive oil. | *Supermarket BBQ sauce.* Tomatoes, garlic, onion, peppers, brown sugar, molasses, special combination of spices and fresh habanera peppers. | *Fast food restaurant BBQ sauce.* Glucose fructose syrup, water, tomato puree, red wine vinegar, spirit vinegar, salt, modified maize starch, vegetable oil (rapeseed), mustard flour, colour (sulphite ammonia caramel), stabiliser (xantham gum), flavouring, preservative (potassium sorbate). |
| **Burger bun** | *Home made bread buns.* 100% whole wheat flour, water, sesame seeds, olive oil, yeast, honey, salt. | *Supermarket burger bun.* Organic sprouted wheat, malted barley, sprouted millet, sprouted barley, sprouted lentils, sprouted soybeans, sprouted spelt, filtered water, fresh yeast, sea salt | *Fast food restaurant burger bun.* Flour, water, salt, sugar, yeast, sesame seeds, rapeseed oil, wheat fibre, soya flour, emulsifiers (mono and diacetyl tartaric acid esters of mono and diglycerides of fatty acids, sodium stearoyl lactylate), palm oil, preservative (calcium propionate), flour treatment agent (ascorbic acid) |

## Food Comparison Chart (continued)

| Food | Real Food | Lightly Processed | Fake Food |
|---|---|---|---|
| Ice cream | *Home made ice cream.*<br><br>Frozen fruit | *Supermarket ice-cream.*<br><br>Water, agave syrup, cashew nuts, carob or cacoa powder | *Fast food restaurant sundae.*<br><br>Ice cream: Skimmed milk, cream, sugar, whey powder, glucose syrup, stabiliser (guar gum, mono and diglycerides of fatty acids, nature identical flavouring, carrageenan, dextrose.<br><br>Sauce: condensed whole milk, Glucose-fructose syrup, butter, modified starch (hydroxyl propyl distarch phosphate), malted barley extract, stabiliser (sodium citrate), salt, flavour, flavour vanillin |

# Rule 4: Progress not perfection.

*"What saves a man is to take a step. Then another step."*

*~ Antoine de Saint-Exupery*

It has been said, 'that a journey of a thousand steps starts by taking the first step.' Know that you have already taken your first step towards weight loss simply by reading this book.

Rest assured that upgrading your food choices is very much a journey of progress not perfection.

You may feel that eating 80% real foods from where you are today might not be possible. But if you stay with the process and take small steps towards your goal, substituting fake foods as you go along, then you will certainly be able to create big changes in your body as you make progress in the long term.

It took me a couple of years before I was eating real foods the majority of the time. What made this much easier for me was changing my food focus towards drinking lots of water, fresh juices and smoothies, whilst also eating a wide variety of soups, salads, vegetables and stews.

Even now after being on the path for over 10 years I am not perfect. Nor do I aspire to be. Unlike what the dieting model may have led you to believe, you don't have to be perfect to get amazing results.

The philosophy of 'progress not perfection' is still very much a part of the way I eat today. I find that it gives me the flexibility to enjoy and experiment with food as well as my life.

In the beginning, you will certainly try things that just won't work for you. That is okay. You don't have to get it right first time. Your body is very forgiving.

Just know that every step that you take is an opportunity to develop deeper awareness and understanding about yourself.

**Breaking free of perfection.**

The dieting industry creates a false expectation of perfection that is simply unrealistic and unattainable for most women.

Melissa, a client I was working with from New Zealand emailed me saying

*"Katrina, I know I need to fundamentally change my eating and living style for myself but it has to be without triggering my punishing doomed-to-fail-fundamentalist-perfect-solution behaviours."*

I assured Melissa that by adopting a 'progress not perfection' approach to eating, she would be able to relax more around food without triggering her 'perfectionist tendencies'.

Since adopting this approach she has found so much more freedom around food and has been amazed at the ever increasing levels of kindness that she extends towards herself.

**Rebuilding my relationship with food.**

JK Rowling, author of the Harry Potter series famously said *"Rock bottom became the solid foundation from which I rebuilt my life."* In much the same vain, rock bottom was the place that I started to rebuild my relationship with food.

One thing that I discovered is that the only thing my body truly craved was proper nutrition. Eating low nutrient food made it difficult for my body to ever feel satisfied. Given that my body's nutritional requirements were not being met, it was no wonder that I continued to have an insatiable desire to eat. This is why you can still feel hungry even after eating large quantities of fake food.

After my physical break down, I wanted to get a better understanding of the nutritional deficiencies that existed within my body. To achieve this, I had a hair and mineral analysis test done through my naturopath. What this basically entailed was cutting a small clip of my hair and sending it off to a laboratory for analysis. From this hair sample I was given a report that detailed exactly where my body was nutritionally out of balance.

Given that my health had completely broken down I found that this was an excellent place for me to start. Depending on your preferred approach and where you are on your journey you may find that you feel drawn to doing this as well.

Another helpful thing to test for is food allergies and sensitivities. Many women may have food allergies without even realising it. Common food allergies come from gluten, wheat, dairy, sugar, caffeine and alcohol. If you crave these substances, then I encourage you to consider a gentle detoxifying cleanse.

One of the food nuances that I have personally found interesting is how women are often allergic to the foods that they are addicted to. This is particularly the case for women who have high amounts of toxicity within their bodies (we will explore some simple detox tips later on in the book).

**Your body is holistically connected.**

What this process helped me to become more aware of is how the body is intricately and holistically connected. What I didn't realise at the time was that being overweight is a key indicator of nutritional depletion and deficiency.

As hard it was for me to initially comprehend, most overweight people who eat high levels of 'fake foods' are actually malnourished. What this means is that the body is not getting the right type of nutrition or it is not absorbing the nutrients properly.

Having regular tests will help you to keep motivated and on track with your weight loss intentions. I can tell you from personal experience that it is amazing to directly monitor the results that subtle food changes can have upon your body.

**Taking baby steps.**

A fascinating concept that I share regularly in my yoga classes is the power of taking baby steps. Most people falsely believe that success is created by taking giant leaps. My own experience has actually revealed the opposite to be true.

Taking baby steps on your food journey is essential. Trying to change your entire diet overnight may only leave you feeling frustrated, confused and angry. Leaping ahead with radical changes is often not the most sustainable approach to take. You can do extreme things for a short while but they generally won't last. Making radical changes to your food choices are akin to the dieting approach, which simply does not work for most people over the long term.

Give yourself the gift of time to learn about different foods and your new food choices. Creating the right inner and outer environments to support permanent change does take time. Making small gradual changes to your diet over a period of time is the key to changing your eating habits and ensuring your long term weight loss success.

When you make changes to your diet and allow for periods of learning and integration, you will likely find losing weight for good a much easier, enjoyable and sustainable process.

### Each woman is unique.

I spent so many years thinking to myself that if only I could find the right diet book then all of my weight issues would be solved.

I know many women who have devoted much of their lives trying to find that perfect 'one size fits all' approach to eating. I was a victim to this kind of thinking for many years. I remember desperately searching for the 'golden elixir of eating' until I finally came to a very important realisation: It doesn't exist. Everybody is unique.

This is why it is so important that you attune your eating approach to suit the needs of your own body. The food that heals one person might not work for another. Said another way, one persons' tonic may be another persons' poison.

### Be willing to experiment.

Finding ways to eat foods that you like, may involve some experimentation on your part, by adapting the right eating approach. It took me quite a bit of playing around before I found a way of eating that was totally right for me.

By 'right for me' I mean eating in a way that was sustainable and in harmony with my own body. Every woman needs to eat in a way that honours her own body and lifestyle.

Eating right for you takes into consideration your lifestyle choices, beliefs, blood type, body type, religion and food preferences.

To eat right for you, consider the types of foods you like to eat, as well as the foods that you don't like to eat. Eating right for you means eating in a way which appeals to your personal tastes, senses and lifestyle.

## Each experience brings an opportunity for learning.

Each experience, regardless of the outcome, creates an opportunity to learn something new. Let go of the need of trying to get everything perfect. When you accept that getting things perfect or obtaining perfection is not important, you can easily turn your focus towards progress, insight, growth and learning through action.

One way that you can ensure progress not perfection is to upgrade your food choices over a period of time from highly processed, fake foods to real foods. When you upgrade your food choices, your lifestyle decisions and your actions, you can create massive change in your health and your life.

Just keep making small, consistent but regular adjustments to your daily habits and you will begin to experience significant long-term transformation.

## Progress keeps you on track.

Did you know that airplanes are typically 'off course' about 99% of the time, yet most still arrive at their intended destination. How is this possible? The reason why is that the pilot is constantly making adjustments to bring the plane back to its' flight path.

Just like the pilot, realise that going off course is a natural part of your weight loss journey. The secret is to keep going making subtle adjustments as you go along. If you feel yourself go off course, just keep reconnecting back to your intention. Keep aiming for progress and not perfection.

If you do, you will achieve progress and stay on track to achieve your weight loss goals. Creating healthy habits of progress is the key because success is about what you consistently do, rather than the things that you occasionally do.

Keep navigating your way back to simplicity. Experiment with eating different foods and notice how they make you feel. Look for real foods in your supermarket and food shops. Spend time watching documentaries about food and how your food is produced.

**The weight loss journey isn't a race.**

The weight loss journey isn't a race. Enjoy the ride and be conscious that there will be times of frustration as well as joy and elation. Each of these experiences are milestones on your path to healing.

It is important to remind yourself that you have your lifetime to master your habits and create an approach that works for you.

Just keep aiming for progress not perfection as you move towards your health goals. Each day celebrate wherever you are on your weight loss healing journey.

# Measuring your weight loss progress.

Measuring your progress on a weekly or monthly basis can be a great way to keep you motivated and focused on your weight loss journey.

Here are some ways you can monitor your progress.

1. **Have a nutritional test done:** Having a nutritional test done will give you an objective way to monitor and measure your progress. From this initial test you will get an idea of what is happening inside your body, including what vitamins and minerals your body is deficient in as well as those that it is abundant in. Examples of nutritional tests include hair and mineral analysis, blood tests, insulin tests, pH tests, pulse reading, intuitive pendulum dowsing and kinesiology. Enquire with your naturopathic practitioner or holistic doctor and be sure to go back for regular check ups.

2. **Get tested for allergies.** Allergies can be a common cause of unwanted weight retention. If you suspect that your body may be experiencing allergic reactions, it may be another great thing to have checked and monitored.

3. **Buy a bio-impedance scale.** Traditional bathroom scales only measure your weight and can be deceiving. A bio-impedance scale measures the fat, water and muscle mass content of your body and will give you a much better indication of your progress (they range in price from £20 - £50). Just remember that no scale, no matter how sophisticated, will ever tell you how much happier you will feel as you begin to reduce toxicity in your body.

4. **Use your favourite belt or pair of jeans.** A low cost and easy way to track your weight loss progress is to notice your jeans (and belt) becoming bigger as your body shrinks. This is a particularly great way to track your progress if you have an aversion to weighing yourself with the bathroom scales.

# Chapter Two - Exercise

*"Movement is a medicine for creating change in a person's physical, emotional, and mental states."*

*~ Carol Welch*

| The Dieting Approach to Exercise | The Healing Approach to Exercise |
|---|---|
| ✘ Focus on creating physical fitness | ✓ Focus on creating health and wellness |
| ✘ You have to sweat it out | ✓ Honour your body's natural energy |
| ✘ No pain, no gain | ✓ Gentle movement and stretching |
| ✘ Burn calories to lose weight | ✓ Focus on your breath and breathing |
| ✘ You have to push and punish your body | ✓ Nurture and reconnect to your body |
| ✘ Exercise is a punishment | ✓ Exercise is a fun way to move your body |

## Begin with gentle movements.

*"Take care of your body. It's the only place you have to live."*

*~ Jim Rohn*

When many women contemplate what it takes to lose weight they imagine having to squeeze into their workout clothes and sweat it out in the gym, pound the pavement or bounce up and down in aerobics classes.

The idea of having to commit to grueling workouts alongside gym junkies, who already have perfect bodies, is enough to put most women off the idea of exercising for life.

One thing I really want you to understand is that you don't need to run, lift weights or do any form of exercise that you find embarrassing or don't enjoy. There are so many wonderful movement options available to you. It's all about finding a form of movement that you enjoy and works for you.

It is also worth noting that committing to a rigorous exercise program when your body is already under stress can actually end up having the opposite effect to the one you desire. So many women unknowingly gain weight these days due to adrenal exhaustion. Moving your body with gentle movements is a gentle way to rebalance your internal body systems. This approach allows you to heal your body from within.

When I started to lose weight, I wasn't capable of doing any form of sustained exercise at all. Instinctively I felt that physically pushing myself by doing any form of extreme cardiovascular exercise was the worst thing that I could do. I was already physically, emotionally and spiritually exhausted.

Rather than push myself needlessly, my focus in the early stages was on creating the right internal environment for my body to get well. As I began to recover I started paying attention to my body's natural desire to move.

If you are already feeling chronically stressed out, I can guarantee that your body is feeling that way too. Over-riding your body's intelligence and pushing yourself through a demanding exercise routine early on in your weight loss journey, may actually do you more harm than good.

**The best place to start.**

When it comes to moving your body, the place I recommend everyone start is with gentle body movements. This will work especially well if you are working on re-establishing your confidence, trust and connection with your body.

You can begin moving right now without even leaving your chair. Start by taking a nice deep breath in. Gently form your fingers into a loose fist and then allow your whole body to release. What do you notice when you do this? What kind of sensations does this movement give you? Are there any other parts of your body that would also enjoy moving?

At the beginning, there is no need to push yourself or your body. Just start out slowly. Begin gently and extend big doses of kindness to yourself as you do. Encourage yourself with every positive step that you take.

In these early stages it is important that you release any self criticism and judgment that you may have. If you think negative thoughts of criticism like "I should do better" just let them go and affirm something positive to yourself such as, *'I am feeling healthier each day'*.

Another useful thing that you can do to support this healing process is to close your eyes and imagine your body moving with grace and ease.

Visualise yourself feeling comfortable in your own body. With repetition, this feeling will become a natural part of your life (we will cover the power of visualisation in more detail later in the book).

Gentle exercise is the way to begin moving, connecting and healing your body. Keep focusing on subtle movements while you build up your strength, stamina and endurance. Start out moving your body in gentle ways, taking your time. When you are ready, you can choose to step it up by increasing the intensity.

# The power of walking.

*"Walking: the most ancient exercise and still the best modern exercise."*

*~Carrie Latet*

Walking found me quite by accident. One day, after not exercising for quite some time, I suddenly felt a very strong urge to go for a brisk walk. So that's exactly what I did. Much to my surprise, I loved it. I remember getting back home and being in a total state of shock.

My body had never enjoyed the high impact nature of running but I hadn't ever stopped to think that I might enjoy walking instead. Initially, I must admit that I didn't even know if walking counted as exercise. I didn't know if it would help me on my journey of losing weight either because I wasn't pushing myself to 'work up a sweat.'

All I knew was that I just felt better when I walked. It was wonderful to feel so healthy and energised. My walks had the added benefit of helping me create space in my mind. I would often finish my walk with completely new perspectives on my life.

**Step it up with regular walks.**

Over time, I noticed that walking helped me to increase my fitness and change my body shape by helping me to build lean muscle mass and burn excess weight.

Walking is a gentle, soothing and creatively healing form of exercise. You don't need any fancy equipment, you can do it anywhere and at whatever pace you like. And best of all, it's free.

Walking naturally suits the physique of the human body. Walking on a regular basis will build body strength as well as have a positive affect on your emotional well being too.

I started out by walking for just 5-10 minutes at a time and was quickly able to build up to going for much longer walks too.

As your confidence, fitness and connection with your body starts to grow you may like to add in some other more formal movement practices as well.

# Find a form of exercise you love.

*"Me thinks that the moment my legs begin to move, my thoughts begin to flow."*

## ~ Henry David Thoreau

As you progress on the path of losing weight naturally and restoring health back to your body, finding a form of exercise that you love will give you an added boost.

When you find a form of exercise you love, you will transform your relationship to exercise, as well as your body. It is possible to create a loving connection to your body by doing exercise that you enjoy.

To find a form of exercise that you love it is important to spend some time experimenting with activities that you might enjoy. Everybody is different, so the key is to keep exploring with different types of movements until you find a form of exercise that works for you and your body. Just keep reassuring yourself that it is safe to experiment with new styles of movement until your exciting new exercise path is revealed to you.

If you think that you hate exercise, rest assured that you have just not found the right form of exercise for you yet. The human body is designed to move. All you need to do is to continue experimenting. When you find a form of movement that you love, you will know. Something in you will become alive, possibly in a way that you have never experienced before. Once you have connected with this form of activity, consider making it a central part of your life so that you can do more of it.

One of my workshop participants, Henrietta said, *"I am 61 years old and finally I have found a fitness exercise regimen that works for me. I use a skipping rope every morning during the week. Skipping for just*

*5-10 minutes each morning is easy and gives me a great start to my morning. I use a cardiac monitor watch which I can track my progress and it keeps me in my heart rate range. Either winter or summer, I still get at least 10 minutes of intense exercise each weekday."*

Here are 4 tips to help you find a form of exercise you love.

### 1.   Individual or social environment.

If you prefer to exercise alone or in small groups, consider doing yoga, tai chi, chi-gong, golf, rock climbing, skipping, skiing, walking, Pilates, weights or swimming.

If you prefer social activity or being in group environments, consider 5 Rhythms dancing, yoga classes (in a social yoga studio) or joining a sports team.  Often there are many social opportunities in local sports clubs such as tennis, netball, rowing, sailing, basket ball or lawn balls.

### 2.   Competitive or gentle healing environment.

When I was younger I did not enjoy the competitive side of sports.  As a result, I thought that I did not enjoy exercise.  Only later did I find out that it was the competitive side of sport that I didn't like.

What I did discover was that I absolutely loved stretching, moving and connecting back to my body.  As a bonus, I learnt that it is possible to lose weight, create vibrant health and build core strength using gentle forms of movement.

You must match the form of exercise back to your own personality and preferences.  When you do this, you will hit the jackpot.  Exercise will become something that is truly joyful and enjoyable for you.

### 3.   Reflective of your interests and passions.

When movement becomes a part of your life and your lifestyle, it becomes a true expression of who you really are.

So, if you love music, choose an exercise that allows you to indulge your enjoyment of music.  If you love the water, consider body boarding, surfing, wind sailing, scuba diving, snorkeling or going for regular swims in the sea.  If you love adventure, what adventure sports could you participate in?  Consider kite-surfing, jet skiing, parachuting or paragliding.

## 4. Consider the climate you live in.

Pay attention to the climate you live in and choose a suitable form of exercise that you can participate in regularly no matter what weather conditions you experience.

Say for example if you would love to snorkel or scuba dive, but you live in the centre of a land locked country, you will have to reconsider your options. This may provide an opportunity to either move to an area which is more conducive to this form of exercise or choose another type of exercise. You can always do something else and pursue your scuba diving as a holiday passion.

Often your passions can open up to more than just ways to move your body; sometimes they can allow you to step into a whole new way of living and life, if you pay attention and listen.

I have a friend who shifted to a Caribbean Island a couple of years ago. As a result of living on an Island, he is more fully able to spend large amounts of time on the beach, doing what he loves the most; kite surfing, eating tropical foods, being in the sun and swimming in big surf.

Since moving to the Islands, he has naturally lost weight and has never looked happier or healthier. Living in this way suits his approach to life, enhances him as a person and allows him to radiate hope and inspiration to others.

## Discovering yoga.

Whilst walking was the only form of exercise that I used to shed my excess 60 pounds, discovering yoga helped me to keep it off for good.

I fell in love with yoga and the benefits that it offered my life. I couldn't believe that something so gentle could actually be good for me. It didn't feel like exercise at all but rather something that I wanted to do and looked forward to each day.

Yoga has opened up a new path for my whole life. It is not just something that I do to keep fit, but it is something that I do it because I love it. Yoga has become a part of my identity and who I am today.

One of the proudest moments of my life was when I qualified as a yoga teacher. I decided to become a yoga teacher so that I could more fully indulge my love and passion for yoga and also create a great excuse for me to stay fit and healthy. It has created so many wonderful opportunities in my life and I now feel very privileged to be able to offer my 'Yoga and Detox' healing retreats all around the world.

Before I lost weight, I couldn't even imagine myself getting through an entire yoga class let alone develop a regular practice. What I have discovered is that when you find a body movement practice that is right for you, amazing things can happen.

## Connect with your breath.

*"Breathing is the greatest pleasure in life."*

*~ Giovanni Papini*

Breathing is one of the most incredible healing tools there is. It is often over looked as a healing tool because it may seem too obvious or simplistic. But do not let this deter you.

For centuries, breathing has been used as a tool to activate states of bliss and even reach enlightenment. Even if personal enlightenment is not what you are looking for, simply breathing deeply on a regular basis will assist you to look and feel great.

When you fully connect with your breath, you have the chance to reconnect back to your body and yourself. By simply following your breath, you can start to step on the path of health, harmony and healing.

**Breathing properly helps relieve stress.**

Breathing properly will help you to relax and de-stress from worry, anxiety and fear. Reducing stress is a great way to alleviate the desire for emotional eating (more on this later). Remember that relaxation is the true antidote to stress. Darkness disappears in the presence of light. Stress disappears In the presence of relaxation and deep breathing.

There are many ways to learn how to breathe properly in a way that relieves stress and clears old emotions. You can begin to explore the simple power of your breath through meditation, yogic breathing (also called pranayama), yoga nidra (a form of guided relaxation) or any form of relaxation that encourages proper breathing. This promotes deep healing and restoration through breathing.

In my yoga classes I like to share with my students the importance of proper, deep belly breathing.

Taking a breath is the first thing you do when you arrive on planet earth and the last thing you do before you leave. Most of your breaths in between go unnoticed.

When you bring your conscious awareness to your breath in the present moment, you will realise that it is the only thing you ever need.

Regardless of what is happening in your life, know that when you simply connect to your next breath, everything is going to be okay.

**Breathing and meditation.**

Meditation is a powerful way to connect with your breath. Breathing can help you attain deep states of relaxation.

There are many styles of meditation including Transcendental Meditation (TM), breath watching, walking meditation and empty mind meditation. Each type has a different energy and texture. If you are keen to experience the benefits of meditation, try out the different styles until you find one that you really love and enjoy.

Meditation can be varied according to your personal preference. Meditation can be done alone, in a group, in silence, chanting or with music. Meditation can be done while sitting down, lying down, walking on the beach, seated on a bus, waiting in a line or in the comfort of your own home.

Meditation is like a pause button; it helps to slow everything down so that you can become conscious and present. It is consciousness that brings a sense of awareness to the things that truly matter. This distinction can help you to let go of unimportant things and bring your mental attention and focus to what really counts in your life.

**Each breath has two distinct parts.**

Within a full breath there are two distinct parts; (1) inhalation and (2) exhalation.

(1) Inhalation

When you breathe in, stop and consciously think about what you are doing. Notice and observe the oxygen move in through your nose and down into your chest. Consider that within this one breath you are literally breathing in 'life-force' energy.

This time notice what happens inside your body when you breathe in. Can you feel your whole upper body move? Your lungs expand, along with your diaphragm. Take your attention all the way to your naval and breathe deeply all the way down into your belly. Allow your belly to expand.

Many women unconsciously breathe in a shallow way, usually only breathing into their chests. The proper way to breathe is to inhale in through the nostrils, breathing all the way down into your naval.

If you watch a baby breathing you will see that their breath naturally expands their lungs and belly too. Try putting your right hand over your belly button and keep inhaling until your hand moves. Feel the natural expansion in your lungs and belly with each in breathe.


(2) Exhalation

Allow your mind to relax as you breathe out. Release everything. Just let your breath go. Feel your lungs deflating and your whole body relaxing. With awareness, let go of any tension or tightness currently stored in your body; maybe your shoulders, your mind or even your jaw. Soften everything as you breathe out. A lovely thing that you can say to yourself as you exhale is, 'It's safe to let go.'

Breathing properly fuels your brain, as well as your body. The oxygen you are inhaling acts as invisible food for your whole body; revitalising your muscles and your organs by oxygenating your entire blood stream.

As you re-energise through the breath your body will feel invigorated. Breathing has the added benefit of reconnecting your body, mind and spirit.

# Chapter Three - Body

*"Our bodies communicate to us clearly and specifically, if we are willing to listen to them."*

*~ Shakti Gawain*

| The Dieting Approach to the Body | The Healing Approach to the Body |
|---|---|
| ✗ The body gets it wrong and makes mistakes | ✓ The body is infinitely intelligent |
| ✗ Don't listen to the body, science has the answers | ✓ Listen to the body and ask, 'What is it communicating?' |
| ✗ The body needs drugs, pills or surgery | ✓ The body has the ability to self heal |
| ✗ Attack and target 'problem' areas where fat is stored in the body | ✓ Create a loving, honouring and respectful relationship with the body |
| ✗ Excess weight is the problem | ✓ Excess weight is the symptom |
| ✗ Fat is to be removed and even cut out of the body | ✓ Fat protects the delicate internal organs of the body from high levels of toxicity |

## Your body is your barometer.

*"Within my body are all the sacred places of the world and the most profound pilgrimage I can ever make is within my own body".*

*~ Saraha*

Your body is the ultimate barometer and feedback mechanism of how you are living your life. Your body is always talking to you, but are you listening?

Your body is created from the air you breathe, the fluids that you drink and the food that you eat. To perform optimally it requires fresh air, clean water and nutrient dense whole foods; high in antioxidants, enzymes, vitamins and minerals.

Carrying excess weight is a clear signal from your body that something is out of balance and needs attention. Excess weight is often a message from your body that it wants less stress and toxicity and more nutrition, rest and relaxation.

Your body is constantly sending you messages and guidance on how to restore your energy and balance. The trouble for many women with weight problems is that they have become disconnected from the natural guidance of their bodies. As a result, when their body speaks to them, they have trouble hearing and recognising the messages it sends.

### The problem of over riding your body.

When you over ride your body's inner wisdom you create internal stress. This stress left unattended for prolonged periods of time, can result in excess weight gain and may also lead to many other chronic conditions.

Your body will communicate with you softly at first, just like a gentle tap on your shoulder. If you keep overriding your body, the messages will start to get louder and more insistent. If left unaddressed they can ultimately end up in some form of a serious wake up call.

Wake up calls are your body's last ditch attempt to get you to pay attention and restore balance in your life. These calls can come in the form of physical, mental or emotional break downs, chronic health problems and in extreme cases, near death incidents.

This is exactly what happened when my own body broke down. I had been overriding my body's inner wisdom for so long. The gentle messages my body had been sending me were being ignored. It was time for my body to get my attention.

Typical examples of how you may be overriding the gentle messages of your body include:

- Saying yes to things you really want to say no to.
- Going out with your friends even when you are exhausted.
- Skipping meals whilst under time pressure.
- Looking after the needs of your partner or family members whilst neglecting your own.
- Working longer hours than you really should.

**Putting everyone else first.**

One of the biggest problems I see women encounter on the weight loss healing journey is putting the needs of everyone else first.

Women are notorious for putting their husband, partner, children, families and even careers ahead of their own needs. From times of early civilisation, women have been the main nurturers within their family unit and communities. Fulfilling this important role can often come at the expense of looking after their own personal needs.

If you are someone who puts your needs behind others, realise that this strategy will often result in you experiencing burn out. Subordinating your own needs is a harmful pattern that makes it extremely challenging to create long-term health. Losing weight is a journey to recognising and acknowledging your own true worth. Placing your own needs first is an important part of this process.

Have you ever wondered why airlines ask you to fit your own oxygen mask first in their safety demonstrations? Well there is a very good reason for it. Being unable to breathe yourself makes it very difficult for you to help or attend to the needs of anyone else. Just as you are asked to always fit your own oxygen mask on an airplane, it is essential that you put your own needs first if you are serious about creating sustainable health within your body and losing weight for good.

One client I worked with thought that it was incredibly selfish to put her own needs first. This was a reflection of how she perceived herself and her own value. She created her self worth from doing things for other people. Her attitude also explained why she was overweight, always late for meetings and generally running behind on things in her own life. By reorganising her priorities and putting her own needs first she found that she was then able to give so much more to others and herself.

If you want to restore health and lose weight for good it is imperative that you start putting your own needs first. When you look after your own needs first, you will be in a much better space to be able to serve your family, friends and community.

**Your body's unique language.**

Just as you have your own unique fingerprints, your body also has its own unique language.

Learning how to understand and interpret your body's language is an essential part of your self-discovery and healing. As you start listening to your inner guidance, you will be able to hear it guiding you towards optimal health and wellness.

Learning to listen to your body can be like learning a new language. At first it will sound like 'gobbledygook'. If you continue to listen to the language, you will begin to hear words that stand out and then also begin to recognise entire sentences and phrases.

If you keep practicing the art of listening to your body you will eventually become fluent in understanding your bodies' unique form of communication.

**So how does your body communicate to you?**

Your body communicates with you via your senses using its own sensory language. This communication naturally filters your thoughts, emotions and feelings. It can also provide physical feedback (via your skin, your hair, your tongue, your eyes and also through your energy levels). You can experience this through feelings of health, dis-ease, happiness, sadness, tiredness, pain, exhaustion, addictions and even food cravings.

How your body works (or doesn't work) can tell you so much about your life and how you are living it. When you receive a message, pay attention to it and then use it to make necessary adjustments to your life.

Your intuition is also a great tool to help you interpret what your body is trying to say. The more you listen to and trust this guidance, the clearer the messages will become.

When you listen to your body it will teach you so much. Just as a mother can learn how to distinguish between the different cries of her baby, with practice you too can learn how to understand and interpret the different messages of your body. Just keep listening to your body and allow it to be your teacher and your guide.

Learning how to listen to your body can take time, so be patient. Keep paying attention to what is happening around you, especially when you experience particular feelings on a recurring basis.

Realise that your body is infinitely wise beyond the realms of your conscious mind. Just by being truly grateful that you have a body can often be enough to place you on the path to healing and losing weight permanently.

**Respect your body.**

Being overweight is a clear message from your body that it wants to be treated differently. If you are like most women, you probably weren't taught how to honour and respect your body as you were growing up.

To honour and respect your body means to treat it with love, gratitude and appreciation for all that it does for you. Astrid Alauda, says *"your body is a temple, but only if you treat it as one."*

If you place a flower in fertile soil and provide it with the right amount of sunshine and water, then chances are it will flourish. Take the same flower and put it in soil devoid of nutrients, without adequate sunshine and water and it will wither and die.

If you are not currently respecting and honouring your body in a way that you like, then realise that with awareness this is something that you can change. Trust that life has brought you to this moment so that you can heal your body and more fully appreciate yourself.

When I run yoga classes I find that for some women it is the first time that they have been able to deeply connect to their bodies, beyond their head and shoulders.  One student told me that in the class she had a deep realisation that she had spent her entire life living from her head, with absolutely no awareness of the needs of her body.  Another student told me that she was more fully able to appreciate her body and the work that it did for her.  With these deeper insights they realised that now they wanted to begin looking after themselves.

**Your body speaks your truth.**

On the journey of losing weight for good, it is important to recognise that your body is your friend.  It is there to support your desire to be healthy and happy.

The way it does this is by always speaking your truth.  Your mind can trick you and even lie to you by the way it rationalises things.  Your body on the other hand, is pure in its' intent to express your inner truth.

# Listening to your body.

You can listen to your body by observing and noticing the feedback that it gives you.  When you first begin to decipher you body's messages, it can pay to do so under the guidance of a holistic Doctor or natural Health Practitioner.  Common things to pay attention to include:

1. **Energy levels:**  Do you feel refreshed and alert when you awaken or do you still feel tired?  Do you need a coffee to 'wake' you up?  If so, you may be nutritionally depleted and in need of an extended period of rest.  Try increasing your nutrient intake, going to bed earlier and reducing or eliminating stimulants such as caffeine, gluten, chocolate, sugar and alcohol.

2. **Hunger and thirst levels:**  If your appetite for food and water is not regular then it could mean that you are disconnected from your physical needs.  Try eating and drinking at regular intervals and using gentle movement practice such as stretching and yoga to help reconnect your body and mind.

3. **Urine colour:** Your urine should be a clear, pale yellow colour. If it is darkly coloured or has an unusual odour, you may be dehydrated or have a urinary tract infection.

4. **Bowel movements:** Bowel movements should be regular. Things you can do to improve your bowel include: eating more vegetables, exercising lightly after eating, gently massaging your stomach, taking supplements such as digestive enzymes and probiotics or going for a series of colonics.

5. **Sickness, illness or disease:** Any form of sickness is a message that something in your body is out of balance. Work with a health professional to find out what you can do to restore balance again.

## Self heal through detoxification.

*"The best way to detoxify is to stop putting toxic things into the body and allow it to depend upon its own mechanisms."*

## ~ Dr. Andrew Weil

Cleansing and detoxifying your body is a great way to activate your body's self healing abilities. It will give your body an incredible feeling of health and wellbeing whilst helping to bring your body back into balance; physically, mentally and emotionally.

With our fast-paced modern lifestyles most women unknowingly suffer from high levels of toxicity. Toxins are everywhere. You will find toxins in the food that you eat, the water you drink, the air you breathe and the pharmaceutical medications you take. Even excess stress can have a toxic affect upon your body's internal health.

This may appear disturbing. The good news is that your body comes fully equipped with the natural ability to eliminate toxins from your system. The challenge arises however when your body's internal elimination system becomes overburdened, so that it cannot cope with the toxicity levels it is being exposed to.

One way that you can help your body to release these excess toxins is by following a cleansing and detoxification protocol. This will help your body to begin the natural process of self healing. Cleansing and detoxifying your body brings it back to harmony, health and balance.

**So how can you tell if your body is toxic?**

When your body is out of balance, then chances are it has become over-burdened with excess toxicity. Your body speaks to you by exhibiting symptoms of being unwell which includes holding on to excess weight. This is why it is important to listen to your body and give it the opportunity to cleanse itself through detoxification.

What most women do not realise is that fat is simply stored toxicity. To deal with high levels of toxicity, your body creates a protective layer of body fat to 'wrap' around the toxins. This protects your vital organs from the poisonous and dangerous effects of toxicity. When this occurs your body will store the toxins in your body to be cleared and detoxified at a later stage.

**Ways to detoxify your body.**

There are many ways to detoxify your body. Two common ways that your body naturally eliminates excess toxicity are via your liver and your skin.

When my body broke down, my naturopath suggested that the best thing for me to do was to detoxify my body, starting with my liver. She told me that my body would be able to heal itself once my liver was functioning and well.

When I began to lose weight, I focused on one thing: reclaiming back my health and life force energy. Little did I know that by cleansing my body I would begin to lose weight at the same time.

Below are some simple steps to help you get started on the detoxification process.

**Simple ways to start detoxifying your body.**

There are some very simple things you can do to help your body naturally cleanse and detoxify.

**1. Drink lemon water:** One of the best and easiest ways to help your body with the cleansing process is by beginning each day with a big glass of lemon water. Your body loves water. Water is a catalyst for cleansing, detoxification and self healing. Lemon juice is naturally alkalising. Drinking lemon water can help your body to naturally and gently kick start the cleansing and detoxification process.

Making lemon water is simple. All you need to do is pour yourself a big glass of filtered water and squeeze in the juice from ¼ of a fresh lemon. Drink it on an empty stomach. I drink my lemon water first thing in the morning upon waking, half an hour or so before I eat breakfast.

**2. Eat detoxifying foods:** Another easy and simple way to help your body with the cleansing process is by eating plenty of detoxifying foods during the day. Grapefruits are a great, natural food that can help to detoxify your body. They make a tasty breakfast or healthy snack during the day. Other powerful detoxifying foods are fresh fruit and vegetables such as beetroot, carrots, parsley, watermelon, apples, blueberries, watercress, garlic and turmeric.

**3. Drink freshly squeezed juices:** A great way to incorporate more fresh vegetables and fruit into your diet is through drinking fresh fruit and vegetable juices. There are 2 types of micro nutrients that your body needs to function optimally; vitamins and minerals. Drinking fresh vegetable and fruit juices are an easy and tasty way to boost your vitamin and mineral nutrient intake.

**4. Use a skin brush:** In your daily shower, gently brush your skin with a natural body brush, available from any health food store. This encourages your body to eliminate toxins out through the pores of your skin, as well as activating your lymphatic system. The skin is responsible for approximately 25% of the body's detoxification each day, which makes it a great way to eliminate toxins from your body.

**5. Practice deep belly breathing:** Breathe fully using your belly. Breathing properly helps to release toxicity. You can assist toxicity elimination through deep belly breathing. This type of breathing engages your tummy muscles and uses the full capacity of your lungs.

Adding these daily rituals into your life is a great way to give your body the support it needs to cleanse and naturally detoxify itself. These simple, cleansing and detoxification rituals greatly assisted me to lose weight naturally and they will work for you too.

**Working with the effects of detoxification.**

As you begin to detoxify your body you may experience 'detox symptoms'. These can be triggered when you withdraw from a regular chemical substance such as gluten, sugar, coffee, tea, chocolate or alcohol. As you begin to detoxify, large amounts of old toxins are released from your body and dumped into your blood stream for elimination.

The more toxic your body is, typically the more detox symptoms you will experience. These symptoms are unique to each person depending upon how toxic they are. What this means is that during the process of detoxification, it can be common to feel much worse before you feel better.

When I run my 'Yoga and Detox' retreats I regularly ask people to share how they are feeling as they progress throughout the week. The variation in detox symptoms is incredible, ranging from 'feeling nothing different' to 'feeling emotional' to having 'a headache or even experiencing mild 'cold-like' symptoms.

If you do experience any detoxification symptoms know that this is a good sign. The best thing to do is to rest, drink plenty of water and let the detox symptoms pass. Typically they pass within a day or two.

# Detoxify and hydrate your body with water.

Providing your body with adequate fresh water is essential so that your body can begin the process of natural detoxification, weight loss and restoring optimal health to your body.

Your body needs water to flush out toxins as well as cleanse and heal itself. It also keeps your body internally moisturised, enhancing cellular activity and body function.

Many people know that they must drink water, but how much is the right amount to drink?

Recognise that every 'body' is different and that your own water needs will vary according to your personal lifestyle.

The best way of revealing the perfect amount of water for you is to listen to your body. Start out by drinking 1 to 2 litres of water a day, filtered if possible. After you make these changes, observe how you feel. Let your body be the guide to the exact amount of water you need.

Hydrate your body with water by using these body messages as your signs:

1. If you feel thirsty, know that you are probably already dehydrated. See if you can drink water throughout the day, to prevent dehydration. Constant thirst can be a sign of chronic dehydration.

2. Notice what other messages your body is sending you. For some people signs of dehydration can include headaches, constant thirst, food cravings, dark yellow urine, waking up thirsty in the middle of the night or being thirsty upon waking in the morning.

## Rest your body.

*"Sometimes the most urgent thing you can possibly do is take a complete rest."*

*~ Ashleigh Brilliant*

Resting your body is an incredibly important part of restoring balance to your body and losing weight naturally. Resting includes making sure that you have personal relaxation time each and every day as well as adequate sleep.

Deep rest and relaxation is the anti-dote to stress and exhaustion. When you are feeling run down, your body can be rejuvenated naturally when you give it the rest that it desires.

In our busy and demanding 21$^{st}$ century living; napping, sleeping and resting are one of the first things to be overlooked or compromised. When I teach my workshops and yoga retreats in Mediterranean countries, it is wonderful to see that many locals still observe an afternoon siesta from 2pm – 5pm.

Quality sleep plays a critical role in creating health and happiness in your life. Sleep is an essential part of healing and rejuvenating your body and will also help you to shift those extra pounds.

Even though you are sleeping, your body is still working hard for you. It is in these moments of resting when your body undergoes deep healing through cellular detoxification, repair and renewal. Interrupted sleep patterns interfere with this natural process and can adversely affect your long term health.

Science is still learning much about the correlations between lack of sleep and weight gain. A study conducted by the National Sleep Foundation found that Americans sleep an average of two hours less than they did 100 years ago. It is believed that sleep deprivation is one of the key factors in the alarming increase in obesity rates. There also appears to be a strong correlation between sleep deprivation and increased appetite.

Before my body broke down, I was constantly pushing my body to the limit. I traded my precious sleep for a lifestyle of studying and working during the day and socialising into the early hours of the morning.

To compensate for my chronic lack of sleep, I would over stimulate my body with excess caffeine, chocolate and sugar. To make matters worse, when it was finally time to rest, these stimulants would end up interfering with the quality of my sleep as well. It was a perfect cycle of unhealthy living.

**Becoming conscious of your sleep patterns.**

If you feel out of balance; physically, mentally or emotionally, then it is definitely worth taking a closer look at your sleeping patterns.

Do you dream of sleeping in? Do you wish you could go on holiday just to 'catch up on sleep'?

If you feel run down, exhausted or feel as if you could 'sleep for days', then there is a high probability that you are deficient in sleep.

Listening to this urgent feedback from your body is the first step to changing your lifestyle and indeed your life.

'Sleep debt' is a problem that many women unknowingly suffer from. It can be akin to debt being accrued in your bank account. At some stage it must be looked at and addressed before things get out of hand. Women who are most prone to 'sleep debt' are women who are stressed and over exerted. Oftentimes, it is only when you stop to catch up on sleep that you realise how big your 'sleep debt' really is.

As crazy as it may sound, booking your own personal 'sleeping holiday' could be exactly what you need to start restoring balance back to your body. Afternoon naps and short breaks are another way to catch up on missed sleep and to bring rejuvenation back to the body.

Interestingly, when my body broke down, the one thing that it needed more than anything else, was sleep. During my recovery period I could comfortably spend up to 16 - 20 hours a day sleeping.

**So how much sleep is enough?**

Again the key here is to listen to your own body. Some people need more sleep than others, so try out a little experimentation and allow your own body to guide you to how much sleep you personally need to create vibrant health.

If you are having trouble hearing clear messages from your body, then try cutting back on things that may be over stimulating you such as coffee, sugar, processed foods, alcohol, surfing the internet, cell phone use and watching television.

If you are still having problems regulating your sleep then it may be worth consulting a natural sleep therapist.

## Reconnect your body-mind.

*"Each patient carries his own doctor within him. The patients come to us not knowing that truth. We are at our best when we give the doctor that resides within each patient the chance to go to work."*

*~ Dr Albert Schweitzer.*

Your body and mind have been designed to function together in harmony and balance. Being physically overweight is an indication that your body and mind are disconnected. When this connection moves out of balance it is a powerful sign that something in your life needs to shift so that you can come back to an internal peace and equilibrium once more.

In our demanding modern day world, many women feel trapped in a chronic cycle of having their minds over ride their body's needs. This cycle, taken to its extreme, can often lead to a total disconnection and dissociation from the physical body.

Advancements in modern technology, although providing many benefits, have played a very big role in this process of disassociation.

The introduction of technological devices such as televisions, computers and mobile phones has resulted in our minds being active for much longer periods of time than they ever used to be. This combined with living more sedentary lifestyles, it's no wonder why so many women have trouble 'switching off' and have lost touch with their physical selves.

When I had my physical break down, my body and mind were in a total state of disassociation. It was like having two flat mates live in the same house refusing to speak to each other. My mind, being the more dominant flat mate, dictated how things were to be done to the total disregard of what my body wanted and needed. This scenario could only ever last for so long before my body decided that 'enough was enough'.

The process of restoring alignment to your body and mind begins with the simple awareness that they are indeed connected. With this awareness established you can then go about building a healthy and functional relationship that is honouring of both of these important aspects of yourself.

When faced with making decisions in your life, asking the following two questions can really help:

1. How does my body feel about this?
2. What does my mind think about this?

When your body and mind are in agreement then this is the recipe for moving forward powerfully in your life. However, if they are in disagreement, then you need to find a more honouring arrangement that works for both your body and your mind.

**Respect your limits.**

To restore your body-mind connection you must learn to respect your limits. Over time, if you continue to ignore your body's need for proper nutrition, water and rest, the most likely result will be fatigue, exhaustion and further weight gain.

A great way to begin understanding your limits is by practicing saying 'no' more often. When you over-ride your body's needs, you may find yourself in situations where you feel forced to do things that you don't want to do.

Saying no can be extremely challenging, particularly for women who like to please and keep others happy. Just know that if you want to lose weight for good, it is important that you learn how to set clear limits and boundaries for yourself.

If you don't clearly express your needs and boundaries you are on the path to burn out. Having been there myself, I know that it can take many weeks and months of focused attention for the body to rejuvenate once it has been pushed too far.

If you have never experienced a burn out before, then it is best to take corrective action before you reach this stage. Let go of any attachment you may have of needing to do everything yourself. Give yourself the permission and space just to be you.

Know that it's okay to say no to other people and put your own needs first. In fact, when you express what you feel, you may find that other people also begin to respect and admire you even more.

Restoring your body-mind connection is an act of deep love and kindness to yourself. Know that your body-mind connection can be strengthened at any stage of your life simply by listening, honouring and nourishing all parts of yourself with high quality nutrition, water and sleep. It also helps to place yourself in healthy, happy and supportive environments.

# PHASE 2:

# Heal Your Mind

# Chapter Four - Thoughts

*"Whatever you can do, or dream you can, begin it.
Boldness has genius, power, and magic in it."*

*~ Johann Wolfgang von Goethe*

| The Dieting Approach to Thoughts | The Healing Approach to Thoughts |
|---|---|
| ✗ Excess weight is a lack of will power | ✓ Excess weight is a sign of imbalance |
| ✗ Control greedy thoughts | ✓ Notice and transform unsupportive thoughts |
| ✗ Think mind over matter | ✓ Imagine and visualise your success |
| ✗ Think calories in, calories out | ✓ Think nourishing and healing thoughts |
| ✗ Focus on dieting rules and dogma | ✓ Focus on your inherent inner wisdom |

## Work with your thoughts.

*"Change your thoughts and you change your world."*

*~ Norman Vincent Peale*

If you want to heal your body and lose weight naturally it is important to recognise the power of your thoughts.

Your thoughts affect your health, particularly the ones that you think over and over again. They have a profound impact upon how you feel about yourself and what you are capable of achieving in your life.

Stated simply, think trim, healthy thoughts and you will create a trim, healthy body. Think unhealthy thoughts and you will create an unhealthy body. It was American philosopher Henry David Thoreau that remarked, *"we become what we repeatedly think about"*.

**It all begins with your thoughts.**

If you want to change the results you experience in your life, it is important to understand how you are creating the results in your life with your current thought patterns.

This happens through a 3 step process as outlined below:

1. Your thoughts create your emotions.
2. Your emotions create your actions.
3. Your actions create your results.

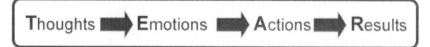

Thoughts ➡ Emotions ➡ Actions ➡ Results

Your thoughts are the catalyst for everything that you experience in your life. If you want to 'change your results', you need to first 'change your thoughts'.

So how long have you been locked into your current thinking? Are your thoughts aligned with what it is that you want to achieve in your life?  Maybe it is time for you to create space for some new thoughts to enter your consciousness?

**Thoughts that harm. Thoughts that heal.**

Think of each of your thoughts as a tiny seed.  If you plant and water a seed there is every chance that it might take root.

'Thoughts that harm' are the seeds of fear and doubt that keep you feeling afraid, confused, unhealthy and overwhelmed.  'Thoughts that heal' on the other hand, are the seeds of your greatness and wholeness.  They fill you with clarity, inspiration, health and happiness.

The good thing is you get to choose which thoughts you pay attention to.  Thoughts attract more of the same thoughts.  If you keep repeating your harmful thinking, then this is what will become your everyday reality.  If you want to heal your body and lose weight permanently, it is important to replace harmful thoughts with healing thoughts instead.

Change starts the minute you begin to work with the quality of your thinking.  Latin writer from 1BC, Publilius Syrus, said it well when he said: *"A wise man will be the master of his mind.  A fool will be its' slave."*

Below is a list of examples of harming thoughts that can be easily replaced with healing thoughts to support your weight loss goals.

| Thoughts that harm | Thoughts that heal |
|---|---|
| 'I am so fat.' | 'I can love my body.' |
| 'I don't know how to lose weight.' | 'I am learning how to lose weight.' |
| 'Losing weight is hard.' | 'Losing weight is getting easier each day.' |
| 'I'll never be able to lose weight.' | 'I can lose weight.' |

| 'I hate my body.' | 'I am learning to love my body more each day.' |
|---|---|
| 'I hate exercising.' | 'I like the way I feel when I move my body.' |
| 'Every time I go on holiday I put on weight.' | 'I come back from my holidays feeling refreshed and healthy.' |

**The power of 'maybe'.**

If you have been trapped in a cycle of harmful thinking and despair, it can take a little time before you permanently switch to a more positive way of thinking.

A simple tool that I discovered for myself to improve the quality of my thinking was the word 'maybe'. Adding the word 'maybe' can break you out of old thought patterns and into new possibilities.

Here are some examples of positive maybes:

- *'Maybe, I can love my body'.*
- *'Maybe, I can lose weight'*
- *'Maybe, losing weight can get easier each day.'*
- *'Maybe, I can love and accept myself.'*

If you can feel your mind fighting your new healing thoughts, just add the word 'maybe' into your everyday language and watch any resistance begin to dissolve.

**Becoming conscious of your thinking.**

I ran a break-through healing session with a nutritionist called Jillian. Being a natural health practitioner, she was well aware what foods she needed to eat in order to create vibrant health. Her challenge however was a seemingly unshakable addiction to cheese and bread that she had only recently developed. She said that these repeated thoughts of 'cheese and bread' would just enter her mind and would demand to be listened to and acted upon.

She told me that she had tried many different techniques to try and control her cravings, none of which had really helped her. Her cravings only seemed to be getting progressively stronger and she wanted to get it sorted before they became totally out of hand.

When I asked her if she could remember when her food cravings began, she told me that they had come on quite suddenly. She explained it to me like this, *"It was as if one day they weren't there and then the next day they were. Every day they seem to get a little bit stronger"*.

As we worked together in our session, one of the things Jillian shared with me was a 'silly fear' she had of growing old alone. Jillian was a successful business woman and had devoted large amounts of time to studying nutrition and building her business. Her dedication had come at the price of not having a whole lot of time left over to build a loving and committed relationship. She said, *"I had always just thought that it would happen when the time was right."*

Jillian had a breakthrough moment when she identified that the cravings were triggered every time she saw 'happy couples' (either in real life or on the television).

Later in our session, Jillian clicked that her cravings began straight after her 40$^{th}$ birthday party.

As we continued to explore, we uncovered one of her unconscious thought patterns which was 'getting old started at 40'. When I bought this to her attention, Jillian quickly added, *"and old people don't find love."* The comment popped out of her mouth, surprising even herself and we both instantly knew that we had uncovered the thought at the base of her cravings.

Jillian was then able to trace the idea back to something that her father used to say. She had taken this on and unconsciously even started to believe it to be true. Once Jillian became conscious of this old and limiting thought program, she was able to see how ridiculous it was for herself.

With this greater awareness of her thinking, she was able to let it go and replace it with more empowering thoughts that supported her goal of finding true love, eating healthily and losing weight.

As Jillian left the clinic room, she told me that she was feeling light and free as a bird. The next day she pulled me aside and whispered that for the first time in a long time that she didn't have any of her familiar cravings for cheese and bread.

She also felt the desire to start up her salsa dancing classes again, clear out most of her wardrobe and start wearing more elegant clothes that flattered her body.

Simply by being willing to investigate her mental thought patterns, Jillian was able to join the dots to make sense of her food cravings and weight gain so that she could address and heal it.

**Working with the unconscious mind.**

The unconscious mind is a very powerful thing and it is important to be aware of how it can take on board seemingly 'ridiculous' thought patterns or ideas.

The thing to be aware of is that your unconscious mind processes every word you say literally. Regardless of what is said, your unconscious mind will accept it as truth.

Each and every word you say really does count. This includes the things you say to yourself as well as others. Interestingly, your mind and body respond as if you are saying it about yourself. When you say to someone else, 'you are so stupid,' your unconscious mind interprets it as 'I am so stupid.'

The other interesting thing is that your unconscious mind does not understand negatives, so even saying "*I am not an idiot*" your unconscious mind processes the statement as if you said "*I am an idiot.*"

Whenever you hear yourself say something negative about yourself or others, just stop and ask yourself how you could restate what you just said in a more empowering and affirmative way. Then say out loud, "*what I really meant to say was...*"

**Change your thoughts, change your life.**

The human mind is full of trickery, illusions and misperceptions. In psychology it is estimated that human beings repeatedly think the same thoughts day after day about 95% of the time. Allowing new and different thoughts to enter your mind is the key to setting yourself free.

Your thoughts are creating your reality on a moment by moment basis. They are the building blocks of your day to day existence. Change your thoughts and you will change your life.

When I was overweight, I was totally unaware about how much impact my daily thoughts were having on my life. It was only after I started to experiment with my own thinking that I was able to see the incredible potential that I had inside of me.

Your moment of power is right now. It doesn't matter how long you have been stuck in your old thought patterns. When you change your thinking, you can start to change your world.

## Move beyond confusion.

*"Simplicity is the ultimate sophistication."*

*~ Leonardo da Vinci*

There is little wonder why so many women feel overwhelmed and confused about losing weight and keeping it off for good. Most top health 'experts' can't even agree on the best ways to lose weight. For every weight loss research study you'll more than likely find another one that contradicts it.

Now I will be the first to admit that the subject of weight loss can be very confusing. It personally took me many years to see through the different smoke and mirror techniques used by the food and diet industry to get people to mistakenly buy their false promises and fake products. There are so many companies that have a vested financial interest in making you believe that something is healthy for you, even when it is not.

The techniques of persuasion and influence used by advertising companies are incredibly sophisticated these days. In the West, we are constantly bombarded with advertisements trying to attract our attention as we make our way through our everyday lives.

Have a good look around you. The 'mislead the customer' approach is used everywhere.

The food industry is notorious for labeling and marketing nutritionally depleted processed foods with buzz words such as 'natural', 'healthy', 'low fat' and 'calorie free' simply to entice consumers to buy their products.

There are companies that are even adding artificial additives, colours and sweeteners to water and then marketing this product as something that is good for you.

**Giving away your power.**

When you are feeling confused, overwhelmed or stressed it is very easy to give your power away. Many companies use techniques to induce disempowered states of being in order to try and get you to 'buy stuff'.

You may be familiar with the following scenario. You open a magazine and it says that the latest research indicates that eating red meat is good for you. It supports its research with impressive looking facts, figures and expert endorsement. So you think, 'Great, eating red meat is healthy and good for me.' Later on, you read another magazine that suggests eating red meat is bad for you with an equally impressive array of facts, figures and expert testimony.

So what are you supposed to do? Eat the red meat or avoid it? Either eating red meat is good for you or it isn't. Surely, it can't be both!

In the past this kind of scenario would make me feel overwhelmed, frustrated and confused. I mean why would one study say that something was good for me and another disagree with it?

**I didn't know what to eat.**

What I found was that the more I tried to listen to 'experts' telling me what was good for my body the more confused I actually became. Living in a complex media driven society, where there are more choices and opinions than ever before, only added to my sense of uncertainty.

With so much conflicting information out there, I wondered how was I ever going to know what to eat? Losing weight just seemed too hard. The more confused I felt the more I would rely on chocolate and other comfort foods for emotional support to get me through the day.

When I was finally able to see that I was never going to be able to find the perfect solution for my body from the outside world, I gave myself permission to find my answers from within.

**Free yourself from guilt.**

One way that you can reduce the amount of confusion you may be experiencing, is to release yourself from any feelings of guilt or obligation.

Every time you say you 'have to do something', you reinforce obligation and confusion within yourself and your life. Realise that there is nothing that you 'have to do'. You don't have to give up chocolate, go to the gym or anything else that you don't want to do.

Here are some examples of words that commonly create confusion, since they are heavily infused with feelings of obligation and guilt:

- *'I really should go to the gym'*
- *'I should watch what I eat'*
- *'I need to go on a diet'*
- *'I need to do more exercise'*

Let these words be red sirens to you and see if you can replace them with different ones. If you choose to let them go, know that you can substitute them with more empowering words such as 'I could', 'I might', 'I can' or 'I am.' Saying 'I choose to' or 'I choose not to' is a much more powerful stance to take.

No one can force you to do anything against your will. You are a free person and can do as you wish. Keep remembering that you always have choices to be clear with yourself and others.

**Navigating your way out of confusion.**

If you want to successfully navigate your way out of the confusion, accept the fact that weight loss can be confusing.

When you become attuned to your body's inner wisdom, losing weight naturally can become an enjoyable journey of self discovery, learning and growth.

Here are some other quick tips to help you navigate your way out of confusion.

- Begin to simplify your life.
- Eat and live as naturally as you can.
- Tune out all the fake promises of the food and dieting industry.
- Take advice from people who have done what you want to do.
- Look for your own answers from within.
- Remember that your body always knows the truth.

## Notice your self-talk.

*"Be impeccable with your word. Speak with integrity. Say only what you mean. Avoid using the word to speak against yourself or to gossip about others. Use the power of your word in the direction of truth and love."*

*~ Don Miguel Ruiz*

If you want to lose weight naturally and permanently, it is essential that you become conscious of your self-talk.

Your self-talk is the ongoing conversation that you have with yourself.

It is the continuous stream of dialogue that spins around in your mind. This voice inside your head provides the running commentary on your life.

When I first became aware of my own self-talk, I was completely shocked when I realised how much mental activity was going on in my mind.

**Why is your self-talk important?**

Peak performance coach, Tony Robbins says that *"communicating with yourself is the most important skill that you will learn in your lifetime."*

The quality of your self-talk sets the tone for how you feel about yourself and ultimately the actions that you are prepared to take in life.

Your self-talk can be your worst enemy or your best friend. The great thing is that it is you that gets to choose.

**Becoming conscious of your self-talk.**

Before you can upgrade your self-talk it is important that you first become conscious of your existing self-talk. Have you ever stopped to think about the quality of the conversation unfolding in your mind? For most people this commentary goes completely unnoticed and unquestioned.

Become aware that you have an inner voice. Do this by acknowledging that this voice is your relationship to yourself. Your self worth and self-confidence are directly affected by it.

I want you to imagine for a moment that there is a special piece of recording equipment that could record all the things that you say to yourself, word for word. Do you think that you might be more than a little surprised when you played back the tape?

Here are a few ideas to help you become more conscious of your self-talk. Simply notice what kinds of things you say to yourself, what tone of voice do you use and if the dialogue is mostly supportive or unsupportive?

**The power of your words.**

Your words are the building blocks of how you see the world. If your words are filled with doubt, pessimism and despair, then this is the way that you will view things. If your words are filled with kindness, integrity and love, then their resonance and vibration will powerfully shape your perception of the world.

When I am working with a client, I pay close attention to the words that they use, the tone of their voice and how they speak. I also observe their body language and facial expressions to see if they are congruent with the words that they use.

Listening in this way gives me a good indication of what is going on in their minds as well as their lives. Tuning into the energy of their words, I am able to quickly ascertain and understand how their current thinking may be causing them unnecessary pain and suffering.

**Pay attention to the words of others.**

It can be challenging to become conscious of your own self-talk, so I generally ask clients to start paying attention to the words of others first. Listen to the words of other people and notice what they say and the impact that it has upon you. Notice whether your feelings change when they use positive and supportive language versus negative and unsupportive language.

Once you have an understanding of the way other people's words affect you, you are in a much better position to become more conscious of how your own language habits and patterns are impacting upon your life. A great way to become conscious of your own words and language patterns is to start beginning to notice:

- How you talk to others
- How you talk to yourself
- How you talk about others
- How you talk about yourself

It is important to pay attention to the things that you say seriously as well as any disempowering things that you say humorously to yourself. An interesting saying that you may have heard before, '*Many a true word is spoken in jest*'.

Words are a powerful tool for activating change and have the ability to transform things positively or negatively in your life depending on how you choose to use them.

**An important word on 'I can't...'**

Have you ever had the experience of making a speech, doing a presentation or completing something that you thought went badly, only to have found out later that someone else thought it was great?

What are you currently telling yourself you can't do?  Whenever you hear yourself say *'I can't....'*, or *'Oh, I could never do that'* allow your inner alarm bells to start ringing.  Just because your mind says something, does not make it true.

Saying *'I can...'* or *'I will...'* or *'I am in the process of...'* is a much more powerful stance to take than *'I can't...'*  From this moment onwards choose to speak to yourself in empowering ways.

Now that you are conscious of it, it will be much easier to notice when it is negative or fearful.  Release the negative, fearful voice by replacing it with life affirming words of compassion, kindness and gratitude.  Know that you can always upgrade your self-talk by speaking kindly to yourself and others.

**Upgrading your self-talk.**

Upgrading your self-talk is the fastest way to build an empowered, loving and healthy relationship with yourself; it is the doorway to connecting to your true self.

Once you are conscious of your thoughts about yourself, then you can begin to take back control of your mind.  Most people have become so accustomed to their inner narrative that they don't even notice it, let alone realise their ability to upgrade it to something more supportive.

## Silence your inner critic.

*"If you hear a voice within you saying, 'you are not a painter' then by all means paint and that voice will be silenced."*

*~ Vincent Van Gogh*

Once you've become conscious of your internal self-talk, one of the first things you will begin to notice is your 'inner critic'.

Your inner critic is the part of you that casts judgment upon your every move. You may experience your inner critic as an unsupportive and unwelcome voice. This voice inhibits your mind, particularly when you start to pursue your dreams.

This internal voice can often have the qualities of an authoritative figure from earlier on in your life, like an unsupportive grandparent, parent, elder sibling, school teacher or friend.

Having a strong inner critic can feel a little like beating yourself with a stick. I know many women unwittingly use their inner critic as a way to motivate themselves. They think that if they can just *'beat up on themselves enough'* then maybe things will change. Let me assure you that there are many more compassionate and effective tools that you can use to create transformation in your life.

Could you imagine if a complete stranger came up to you and started speaking to you in the same way that your inner critic does? I am sure that you would keep walking or possibly even tell them *'where to go!'*

Your inner critic is the part of you that is full of doom and gloom. It is the voice of limitation and fear. For many women, it keeps them small and holds them back from listening to their dreams. It is the inner critic that acts like a victim. It is this part of us that is so keen to tell the story about why 'life is so hard'.

Your inner critic might tell you things such as:

- *'You are not good enough'*
- *'You are never going to make it'*
- *'You will never lose weight'*
- *'You might as well just give up now'*

If any of these comments sound familiar to you, rest assured that you are not alone. The relationship that many women have with their bodies is based on relentless criticism and self-attack. Just know that it doesn't have to be that way particularly when you start to work more effectively with your mind.

**Breaking free from self punishment.**

Several years ago, I had a breakthrough healing session with a young woman called Emma.

In our session together, Emma confessed to me that the first thing she would do every morning after she woke up was to weigh herself. If she weighed 9 stone or less then she allowed herself to eat whatever she wanted during the day with no restrictions. If she weighed over 9 stone, she would berate herself mercilessly and then restrict her eating to nothing but apples, carrots and water for the rest of the day.

She told me that she knew that this wasn't a healthy approach to eating but didn't know how to stop it. Her secretive behaviour had a high cost associated with it. She thought that it held her back from getting what she truly wanted, a loving and supportive relationship.

As the healing session unfolded, Emma was able to see the situation from another perspective and soon even began to laugh about the sheer ridiculousness of it all. By the end of her session, Emma could no longer see any good reason for her self-imposed punishment. We both agreed that given her height, that 10 stone was a more natural body weight for her anyway.

When you work with your mind, you can begin to let go of self judgment and criticism, transforming your relationship with yourself into a much kinder one.

**Turning down the volume of my inner critic.**

This whole area of self criticism is close to my heart because it is something that I personally struggled with for a very long time.

My inner critic was very vocal when it came to offering opinions about my body and my appearance. It was quick to point out everything that was wrong with me. Over time, I ended up being filled with doubts, fears and self hatred for my body. It was like carrying the enemy around inside my head.

I wasn't particularly athletic and found it embarrassing to participate in school sports. Every time I had physical education classes, my inner critic would become active, telling me how fat and useless I was.

When I was overweight, I hated my body. I found it difficult to find clothes that could hide my figure. I thought I was totally abnormal. I didn't look like other girls. My inner critic liked to point out that I had bulging upper arms, a thick neck and was really broad around my shoulders and chest.

Bra fitting was the ultimate in humiliation. As a young teenager, I remember feeling so embarrassed about the idea of going 'bra shopping' with my Mum. I would pull out every excuse to try and avoid it.

I remember standing half naked in the changing room with the shop assistant, imagining all the terrible things she must be thinking about my fat body as she measured me. As it happened, most of the bras that I tried on didn't fit me properly confirming my worst fears: 'there was something wrong with me'.

## My problem was a thinking problem.

As hard as it was to see at the time, I came to understand that my problem actually had nothing to do with my body. My real problem was a thinking problem. It had nothing to do with my size and everything to do with my mind chatter and how I thought about myself.

If you were criticised as a small child, then chances are that you will probably criticise yourself in the same way, even today.

If this is true for you (and from my experience it is with most women), then I recommend that you work with this book and do your inner healing work so that you can break free of your old thought patterns to radically transform the way that you treat yourself.

Changing the way you think about your body, gives you the power to change everything. You can transform the dialogue you have with your inner critic, into something that is more empowering and inspiring.

As you do this on a regular basis the type of relationship you have with yourself will begin to change.

## Making friends with your inner critic.

On my weight loss journey one thing I did for myself was to make friends with my inner critic. This allowed me to alter the relationship I had with myself and my mind.

My inner critic used to speak to me negatively most of the time. It punished me for not being good enough, about practically everything, using words, diets and food as its primary weapons of choice.

I used to think and say things to myself that would have a really negative effect on my self-confidence. I would look in the mirror and say spiteful things to myself, such as: '*I am so fat and useless,*'

Remember that you do not have to believe everything your mind says. Some thoughts will make you feel good. Some thoughts will make you feel bad. Choose to believe the voices that make you feel good.

While I was learning how to be friends with my inner critic, I had to make a conscious effort to ignore my inner critic and pay close attention to the thoughts that uplifted and supported me.

**Silencing your own inner critic.**

Imagine how good it will feel to transform your inner critic into a supportive voice, akin to a best friend.

You can do this. It starts with recognising how powerful your inner critic really is. The time has come for you to get your inner voice to work for you, not against you.

Only you can silence your inner critic. Once your inner voice is trained, it will become a powerful ally on your weight loss healing journey.

Take a moment to connect with your inner critic. Are you willing to transform this voice into something more supportive? With time and practice, you can learn how to soften this voice by gently speaking to yourself with love, encouragement and compassion.

When you feel tempted to mentally beat yourself up, instead find things that you can acknowledge and admire about yourself. As you become more comfortable 'in your own skin' you will be less critical of yourself.

The way I did this was by practicing kindness. Each time I felt like criticising myself, I knew that I could choose words that supported and nurtured me instead.

Learning how to love who you are and becoming fully self-expressed is the key to long term healing and change. When you are ready to heal, know that you can choose to change the way you treat yourself by simply changing your words, thoughts, actions and habits.

**'Thank you for sharing'**

Today I can easily recognise the voice of my inner critic. However, I don't pay it too much attention as over the years, I have learnt not to believe it. I certainly do not listen to what it says. Whenever my inner critic tries to offer me its' opinion I am quick to replace any disempowering or limiting thoughts with positive and empowering ones instead. Here's how I do it...

As soon as I am aware of my inner critic speaking negatively to me, I consciously say to myself, *'Thank you for sharing.'* I repeat this mantra to myself until a new and more uplifting thought or idea slips into my mind. When this happens, my inner critic is silenced and my old, limiting thought quickly dissolves and disappears.

Living in this way enables me to be the master of my own mind. It will also help you to bring your mind into alignment with your health and life goals.

Once you are aware of your limiting thought patterns, then you can break free of them. Realise that they are only thoughts and thoughts can be easily discarded and replaced with new thoughts.

Now is the time to stop the abusive cycle of self punishment that is going on in your own mind. You are a powerful woman capable of being the master of your own mind. Let your mind be your servant and realise that you do have the power to choose what thoughts you decide to listen to and believe.

---

# Exercise: Silence your inner critic.

Take a few moments to listen to your inner critic. In your journal answer the following questions:

1.   What words do you use to scold or criticise yourself?

   .................................................................

2.   When do you criticise yourself the most?

   .................................................................

3.   How could you speak more kindly to yourself?

   .................................................................

# Ask better questions.

*"The only questions that really matter are the ones you ask yourself."*

## ~ Ursula K LeGuin

Learning how to ask better questions is a key aspect of healing your mind and losing weight for good.

As you work with your mind on your weight loss journey, it is important to understand that your mind will always answer any question that you ask. This is regardless of whether the question is a useful one or not.

For example, if you ask yourself the question *'Why am I so fat?'* your mind will do its' very best to come up with plausible reasons why this might be the case. Very often these answers lack the benefit of truth or perspective.

In the past, when I was struggling to lose weight, I used to ask myself questions that led to me feeling bad. This mental battering left me feeling depressed and apathetic. The worse I felt about myself, the more comfort food I sought.

If it is time for you to break free of this cycle of inner turmoil, I suggest that you ask yourself better questions, such as *'How can I lose weight and enjoy the process?'* This will allow your mind to search a little deeper within.

Notice how your mind will always do its best to come up with possible answers to whatever questions you ask.

### Disempowering questions.

I know that many women who experience weight problems fall into the trap of asking themselves disempowering questions that keep them stuck. Most will do this without even realising they are doing so.

When you ask a disempowering question, your mind will come back to you with a stream of reasons about why you can't do something. For example, quite unconsciously it may reply: *'It's because you're stupid'* or *'You are so lazy'.*

Disempowering questions will always lead you to disempowering answers.

**Asking better questions.**

You can easily transform this scenario by learning how to ask better questions. The key is to start getting conscious of the questions that you are already asking yourself.

Once you have achieved this, you can start asking yourself empowering questions that will help move you in the direction of your dreams. If the questions you ask don't help you to do this, start to think of ways you can rephrase what you are asking, until they do. By doing this you will be in a much more powerful and resourceful state of mind to achieve your weight loss goals.

Here are some examples of disempowering questions, with possible replacement questions, for you to study and learn from:

| Disempowering Questions | Asking Better Questions |
|---|---|
| 'Why do I always eat too much?' | 'How can I eat more real foods?' |
| 'Why am I always too tired?' | 'How do I love to move?' |
| 'What's wrong with me?' | 'What great things am I already doing and achieving in my life?' |
| 'Why am I so fat?' | 'What can I do to create health?' |
| 'Why am I such a failure?' | 'Who can help me to succeed?' |
| 'Why do I have no will-power?' | 'Where am I already disciplined in my life?' |

## Getting better answers.

When you ask yourself better questions you will start to get better answers. Your mind will offer you new ideas and possibilities that can help you to achieve a positive outcome for what you want.

The process of asking better questions can be an enlightening one. It will help you to learn more about yourself and what you are truly capable of.

When you speak with powerful and empowering words, your entire being will start to shift. You will respond to your weight challenges differently and you will also attract greater opportunities, people and circumstances into your life.

You will discover new solutions to your challenges that are supportive, encouraging and inspirational. These will assist you on your journey towards healing your body and losing weight naturally.

---

# Exercise: Ask better questions.

Take out your journal and write down your answers to the following questions:

1. Who can support and encourage me to lose weight?

   ............................................................

2. What tools would assist me to lose weight for good?

   ............................................................

3. What is one thing that could help me to lose weight?

   ............................................................

---

## Create healing affirmations.

*"You affect your subconscious mind by verbal repetition."*

## ~ W Clement Stone

An affirmation is a declaration of a state of being or a desired outcome. When stated in the positive it is a powerful tool to assist you on your weight loss healing journey.

Healing affirmations are made up of inspiring words that you can say to yourself, to assist you to achieve your weight loss goals.

Creating healing affirmations for yourself can help you to transform your experience of the present moment as well as shape your future. The most important thing is to make sure that your affirmations are supportive and in alignment with your goals and your dreams.

Nikki, one of my yoga students, uses the affirmation, *'I am the warrior'* to reconnect with her inner strength, focus and determination. She repeats this phrase to remind herself of who she is in the process of becoming.

When you are crafting your affirmations make sure that they are personal, specific and uplifting. They will work best when they are stated in the present tense, evoke a positive emotion within you and are repeated regularly.

When you start using personal affirmations they might feel a little awkward at first. But with constant repetition they will help you to create a whole new reality for yourself.

Affirmations work because they interrupt old or existing mental patterns. When you affirm with conviction and sincerity what you want to create, in time you will attract the resources you need to manifest your desires.

**'A lean, mean, fat fighting machine.'**

When I set out on my weight loss journey, I knew that it was important to take back control of my own thoughts and my mind.

One day I was dreaming about how I might be able to achieve this, when the affirmation *'I am a lean, mean, fat fighting machine'* entered my conscious. When it did, I have to admit that the idea made me laugh out loud. It was a silly thought. But I couldn't help but wonder to myself, *'What if I could be?'*

As outlandish as the thought appeared at the time, it made me feel good and had a healing effect upon the way that I saw myself. So I repeated it in my mind a few more times.

Over the coming weeks I would use the phrase whenever I felt weak or tempted to go back to my old habitual thought patterns. In fact, whenever I affirmed to myself, *'I am a lean, mean, fat fighting machine'* I would instantly feel better. Interestingly, when I thought this, I only wanted to eat nourishing and healthy food.

At the time, I didn't even know what an affirmation was. My understanding of them came much later on. What I did know was that, I was really enjoying the healing effect this short phrase was having upon my mental state of being and self confidence. I began to feel much more powerful and self assured.

I decided to repeat my affirmations to myself on my regular walks. With each step I took, I affirmed over and over again, *'I am a lean, mean, fat fighting machine.'* During my daily walks I repeated my affirmation maybe hundreds of times.

Over time, this affirmation became ingrained into my consciousness. My affirmation would pop into my mind in the shower, while I was driving and even in my dreams at night. It just kept running through my head. With time my affirmation became a part of my new way of thinking and ultimately it shifted the way that I saw myself forever.

During the period of my weight loss journey, if I ever had a moment of hesitation or doubt, I would simply ask myself the following question, *'What would a lean, mean, fat fighting machine do in this situation?'* Immediately the answer would become obvious to me.

You too have the power to shift your focus and perception of the world with the use of affirmations. What would happen in your own life if you could find a simple sentence that would inspire you on your weight loss healing journey?

Feel free to use the affirmation, *'I am a lean, mean, fat fighting machine'* if it works for you. Otherwise create you own personal affirmation in the exercise below.

# Exercise:  Create your own healing affirmation.

Create a healing affirmation for yourself that you can use to give you the focus, strength and determination you desire to achieve your weight loss goals and dreams.  My healing weight loss affirmation is:

........................................................................................................

........................................................................................................

........................................................................................................

........................................................................................................

## Visualise your success.

*"Ordinary people believe only in the possible. Extraordinary people visualise not what is possible or probable, but rather what is impossible. And by visualising the impossible, they begin to see it as possible."*

*~ Cherie Carter-Scott*

When setting out to lose weight naturally it is important that you engage the power of your imagination through visualisation. Visualising your success is a creative process.  Use it to shape a new vision for your life.

Did you know that you are constantly creating your world with the images that you form in your mind on a moment-by-moment basis? Repeated images form the foundation of visualisations.

When I was healing my body and losing weight, I used the process of visualisation to help me.

One day I was imagining the kind of body that I wanted to create. Then I got an idea from a magazine. I wondered, *"What if I stuck a picture from a magazine of a lean, healthy and fit-looking woman by my bed?"*

Again, I laughed at the idea but then I thought, *'I'm going to try it'*. And that is exactly what I did.

Every night before going to sleep and upon waking, I imagined that I was creating my most amazing body using this woman's body as a visual reference.

I visualised my body becoming strong and healthy, just like the woman in the picture. During the day, my mind would reconnect with this picture and I used it to motivate and spur me on to achieve my weight loss goals. This is a powerful exercise as it is aligned with the way that your brain works.

## Engaging your imagination.

The human brain is broken into two hemispheres; a left and a right side. The left hemisphere of your brain is analytical. It processes things using logic and reason.

The right hemisphere lives in possibility. It operates in images and pictures. It fully engages the imagination, both the creative and the spiritual aspects of your being.

When you are creating change in your life, you want to engage the right hemisphere part of your brain as much as possible. This part of your brain sees possibilities in all things. It is holistic, integrative and honours the many different shades of grey between black and white.

Generally, within the Western education system, lessons are taught predominantly using left brain, analytical learning styles such as reading, writing and rote learning.

## The importance of visualisations.

Visualisations are very important because when you use them you are speaking a language that your body can understand.

Repeated images and pictures form your visualisations and your reality. They are powerful because they communicate directly with the unconscious mind (the right hemisphere of the brain) and create a physiological response within the body, affecting your internal body communication and chemistry.

I'll give you an example:

Close your eyes and imagine a ripe and juicy lemon. Now, as you think of this lemon, notice what thoughts, sensations, feelings and associations come over you.

Chances are that you saw a picture of a lemon. You may have even begun to salivate. The reason why all this happens is because your mind works in pictures.

The creation of a picture in your mind of the lemon is enough to create a physiological response.

Thinking about things in this way and visualising them has a direct impact upon your physical body. You can use this simple but profound idea to help you to lose weight naturally.

**Upgrading the pictures in your mind.**

Think about the pictures that you currently hold in your mind. Are they the types of images that will positively or negatively affect you? Will they help you to lose weight? By simply changing the pictures that you hold in you mind about yourself, you can begin to evoke powerful changes to your physical body.

Your outer world is a reflection of your inner world. If you want to transform your experience of your 'outer world', you have to transform what you see in your 'inner world'.

If you want to create health, energy and a healthy body, you need to cultivate the types of images and pictures that will support optimal health, energy and wellness. Health and healing occurs naturally when what you think, what you say and what you do, are all working together in perfect harmony.

# Chapter Five – Beliefs

*"Do not believe in anything simply because you have heard it. Do not believe in anything simply because it is spoken and rumoured by many. Do not believe in anything simply because it is found written in your religious books. Do not believe in anything merely on the authority of your teachers and elders. Do not believe in traditions because they have been handed down for many generations. But after observation and analysis, when you find that anything agrees with reason and is conducive to the good and benefit of one and all, then accept it and live up to it."*

*~ The Buddha*

| The Dieting Approach to Beliefs | The Healing Approach to Beliefs |
|---|---|
| ✗ Dieting is the only way to lose weight | ✓ Focus on gaining health and wellbeing. |
| ✗ Losing weight is hard | ✓ Losing weight is easy when you know how |
| ✗ Follow rules and dogma | ✓ Follow your body's wisdom |
| ✗ Diets equal deprivation and restriction | ✓ Healing equals awareness and growth |
| ✗ Focus on the word can't | ✓ Focus on the word can |

## The role of beliefs.

*"The thing always happens that you really believe in; and the belief in a thing makes it happen."*

*~ Frank Lloyd Wright*

Your beliefs have an important role to play in either helping or hindering your progress on your weight loss healing journey.

A belief is a strongly held conviction that something is true or real. Your beliefs are the filter through which you see and make sense of the world around you. They create your focus and determine what you do and do not pay attention to. Your beliefs are important because they influence the way that you think and the actions that you take in your life.

You can hold beliefs about anything. This includes your body, your state of health and even your ability to lose weight.

### How are beliefs formed?

Your beliefs begin to form during early childhood (between the ages of 2 and 7 years old) and as such are largely influenced by the prevailing assumptions of your family, friends and cultural traditions in favour during this time.

Most of the beliefs that you acquired during childhood are stored within your unconscious mind. Although these beliefs may have served a very real purpose during your formative years, they can and do become outdated as you grow older.

Let's use an illustrative example. When you were young, like most children you were probably told not to talk strangers. Now to a young child this piece of advice can help to ensure their safety and wellbeing. However as a child matures into adulthood, the belief that it is not safe to talk to strangers can restrict the flow of connections, opportunities and overall enjoyment of life.

As you get older, it is natural for your early beliefs to become outdated. With greater life experience, you will be exposed to different perspectives as well as being able to call on enhanced levels of skill, ability, education, resources and life experience.

Your expanded 'tool kit' means that you are better equipped to deal with and handle a wider array of challenges, dilemmas and situations.

Your beliefs about weight loss can be broken down into two distinct categories: '*limiting beliefs*' and '*supportive beliefs*'.

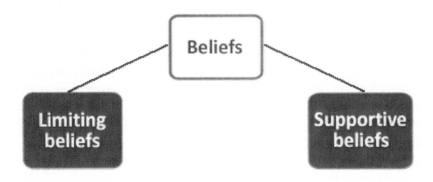

**Limiting beliefs.**

Limiting beliefs hold you back from achieving your goals and aspirations. They are what stand in the way of you achieving your full potential. It is these beliefs that keep you playing small.

Limiting beliefs are especially powerful when they are repeated and engrained until eventually they are accepted as truth. Your limiting beliefs are what hold you back from living life on your own terms and can become a major obstacle to you losing weight and living a healthy and vibrant life.

Examples of common limiting weight loss beliefs include:

- *'I can't lose weight'*
- *'I'm too old to lose weight'*
- *'Weight problems run in my family'*
- *'I've got big bones'*
- *'I hate my body'*
- *'I am ugly'*
- *'I'll never be healthy'*
- *'My energy is not what it used to be'*

If you are experiencing challenge in any area of your life, (whether it be with your weight, health, finances, career or relationships) it is very likely that this could be due to the presence of a limiting belief. When you clear a limiting belief and replace it with a new and more empowering one, you literally transform what is possible in your life.

To lose weight for good, it is essential that you neutralise your 'limiting beliefs' by transforming them into 'supportive beliefs'.

### Supportive beliefs.

Supportive beliefs, on the other hand, aid and assist you in the achievement of your goals and aspirations. When your weight loss beliefs are supportive and in alignment with your goals, long term sustainable weight loss can be achieved.

The more limiting your beliefs are, the more frustrating your life will be. The more helpful and supportive your beliefs are, the more miraculous your life will be.

### Taking off the blinkers.

Take a moment to imagine blinkers on a horse. When a horse wears blinkers, its' range of vision is severely restricted. With the blinkers on, the horse can only see directly in front of it and has no peripheral or side vision.

When the horse wears its' blinkers, much of the landscape it passes is blocked from view. Even though the landscape is still there, with the blinkers on, the horse is not able to see it.

When you hold onto '*limiting beliefs*', you are limited in what you are able to see, just like the horse in our example. When you clear these beliefs you metaphorically 'take off your blinkers' and expand your range of vision for what is possible for you in your life.

### Believe that you can lose weight.

If you want to lose weight for good it is essential that you believe that you can do it. It is also important that you have a willingness to transform your limiting beliefs into supportive beliefs.

Your current weight loss beliefs are an amalgam of your past life experience and what you hold to be true. If you don't believe that you can lose weight yet, at least stay open to the possibility that you can. Even if you have struggled with your weight your entire life, you can create weight loss beliefs that support you in creating a new body and life for yourself.

Always remember that your past is your past. With new empowering thoughts you can create new beliefs that truly serve the person you are in the process of becoming.

When you believe that you can heal your body and lose weight naturally, nothing will stand in your way. Your mind will constantly be on the lookout for evidence to support your beliefs. Even the largest obstacles will not prevent you from achieving success.

Even if you experience setbacks, know that they are only temporary and a great opportunity to further develop your internal strength and character. Believing that you can lose weight is part of knowing that you are worthy and fully deserve to live the life that you dream about.

---

# Exercise: Identify your limiting beliefs.

The contemplation below will help you to identify your limiting beliefs. For each question below, write down the first thought that comes to your mind.

1. My body is

   ................................................................................................

2. Healthy food is

   ................................................................................................

3. Losing weight is

   ................................................................................................

---

## Question your limiting beliefs.

*"Your events, your lives, your experiences, are caused by your present beliefs. Change the beliefs and your life changes."*

*~ Seth*

An essential part of upgrading your limiting weight loss beliefs is learning how to question them. The key thing to remember is that your beliefs are much more flexible than you think. With willingness and awareness they can be easily transformed and updated for the better.

Questioning your health and weight loss beliefs on a regular basis, will help you to reshape your thinking so that you can move beyond your current weight challenges.

### How to question your beliefs.

To ensure that the beliefs that you hold are relevant and in alignment with your goals, it is important that you learn how to question them effectively. Given the wide array of weight loss beliefs that most women hold, you might be wondering about how to start questioning your own beliefs.

The general advice that I give to my clients is to work on a 'needs to' basis. By 'needs to' I mean, if you have a belief that is currently causing you some kind of pain, suffering or anxiety then it is worth taking a closer look at it.

Questioning your limiting beliefs works best when you have a willingness to think new thoughts about your life. This will help you to gain a deeper understanding about yourself.

### Questioning your 'limiting weight loss beliefs'.

If you want to clear a limiting weight loss belief, you need to create doubt in your mind about its truth and relevance.

A simple way you can do this is by asking yourself the following two questions: (1) *'Is this belief true?'* and (2) *'Is this belief helpful?'*

Allow us to work through an example. Let's just say that you hold the limiting belief that 'it is impossible to lose weight' and you've made the decision that this belief is no longer serving you.

### (1)  Ask yourself, 'Is this belief true?'

The first thing you need to ask yourself is 'Is this belief true?'

To disprove the truth of this belief, you simply need to find one person who has successfully lost weight.  The evidence of finding one person who has done this will immediately cast doubt over the validity of this belief.  If you can see that it is possible for someone else to lose weight, then it ignites the creative idea that it might be possible for you to be able to do it too.

The more examples that you can find of people who have successfully lost weight, the more unstable this old weight loss belief will become until it eventually crumbles.  Once you have created enough instability around the old weight loss belief to the point where you accept that it is no longer true for you, you may choose to replace it with a more supportive weight loss belief.

In this example, a much more supportive belief might be *'It is possible to lose weight'.*

### (2)  Now ask yourself, 'Is this belief helpful?'

For us to explore the second question, let's just suppose that you weren't successful in either finding a single person who had successfully lost weight or able to disprove this belief by other means.

The second question that you might like to ask yourself is *'Is this belief helpful?'*

It is important to understand that some beliefs are incredibly helpful.  These are the beliefs that you want to hold onto.  The beliefs that you want to clear or release are the beliefs that are a hindrance in your life or are no longer helpful for you in the realisation of your goals and dreams.

So what happens when you apply this question back to the original limiting belief 'It is impossible to lose weight'?  Now assuming that you genuinely do want to lose weight, holding onto the belief '*It is impossible to lose weight*' is not going to be particularly helpful.

Given this, it would be beneficial to upgrade this belief to something that is more helpful. '*Maybe, it is possible for me to lose weight*'.

Once you have created a new belief for yourself, you need to find supporting evidence to fully embed it into your life and way of being, as we will discover later in the chapter.

**Questioning my own limiting beliefs.**

One of the limiting beliefs that I used to have was '*losing weight is hard*'. I also had another closely linked belief to this one that '*change is hard*'.

If you think limiting beliefs often enough, I can almost guarantee you that they will become part of your accepted reality.

Before I was able to release my limiting weight loss beliefs, I knew that I had to question my beliefs and attitudes around change first. Through doing this I made the decision to embrace a more helpful belief that 'change is possible, change is easy, and change is fun!'

I started looking everywhere for evidence to support my new belief, both in my own life and in the lives of others. Interestingly I began noticing many things in my life that I hadn't paid attention to before.

When I changed my limiting belief from 'change is hard' to 'change is possible, change is easy, change is fun!' I realised that my limiting belief was exactly that - a limiting belief. I also discovered that, with a little focused effort, this limiting belief could be easily replaced with a more supportive belief. With this new awareness, empowering change became not only possible in my life, but highly probable.

Once I was able to feel excited by the prospect of change, I knew that the time had come to upgrade my old belief that '*Losing weight was hard.*' I decided that my new belief would be '*Losing weight is easy when you know how.*'

I immediately started looking for evidence supporting my new belief.

I was able to find lots of different examples of how my new found knowledge and awareness was making the process of losing weight much easier for me.

Feeling motivated and excited by my initial results, I decided to add in a few more supportive beliefs as well, including:

- *'I can lose weight'.*
- *'I am losing weight'.*
- *'I can achieve my dreams'.*

By working through this process for myself, I came to the realisation that my mind will seek out supportive evidence to substantiate any thought that I believed to be true.

If you believe that healthy food is tasteless, your mind will find evidence to support it. If you believe that healthy food is the best tasting food on the planet, your mind will also be able to find equally convincing information to support that belief as well.

The good news is that you have the power to choose your own weight loss beliefs. So why not chose supportive ones that assist your weight loss, healing and growth? When you have congruency and alignment between your weight loss beliefs and your goals, great things become possible in your life.

**Other useful belief clearing tools.**

Questioning your limiting beliefs is just one tool you can use to clear and upgrade them. There are many other powerful healing tools that you can use as well.

Some of my other favourite modalities that are worth exploring for yourself include: Emotional Freedom Technique (EFT), Hypnosis, Neuro-Linguistic Programming (NLP), High Performance Coaching and Yoga.

## Break free from self sabotage.

*"To overcome difficulties is to experience the full delight of existence."*

*~ Arthur Schopenhauer*

If you are committed to losing weight for good, sooner or later as you move along your weight loss healing journey, you will come face to face with your 'inner saboteur.' Typically this is through the unconscious act of self sabotage.

Self sabotage happens when you override your best intentions in a harmful, destructive or self defeating way. It can often occur when there is either a conflict between your beliefs or when different parts or aspects of your personality are in disagreement.

Indicators of weight loss sabotage may include:

- Eating fake foods.
- Eating foods your body is allergic to, even when you know you shouldn't.
- Spending time with friends that would prefer you to stay overweight.
- Staying back at work and missing your exercise class.
- Eating healthily in public but then binging in private.
- Over-exercising when all your body wants to do is rest.
- Eating or drinking alcohol in excess, even when you know you have had enough.
- Watching late night television instead of giving your body the sleep it deserves.

**Self sabotage is an invitation to heal.**

Self sabotage is an opportunity for you to become more congruent and coherent as a human being. With awareness, this can be done by healing internal conflicts and bringing your beliefs and different aspects of your personality into alignment.

The signs of self sabotage will always be subtle to begin with but will progressively escalate if you continue to ignore them. The Universe always knocks gently to begin with. If you do not pay attention the knocks tend to get steadily louder.

It is not uncommon for people who continue to ignore their patterns of self sabotage to experience freak accidents, be diagnosed with a chronic disease or if serious enough, even endure near death experiences.

As a general rule, the more serious the act of self sabotage, the more urgently your higher self seeks your full and undivided attention. It can be easy to blame self sabotage on external events, situations or other people, but in doing this you give away your true power to make affirmative changes in your life.

Self sabotage is calling you to become conscious of the role that you play in the unfolding events of your life. When you are ready and willing to move out of victim mode and take responsibility for yourself, you will begin to see where your unconscious beliefs and thoughts are out of alignment with the person you are in the process of becoming.


**Sabotaging myself.**

In the years leading up to my body break down, I was running an intense self sabotage program that was destroying my life.

Looking back, I realised that I experienced many gentle 'taps on the shoulder.' These warnings urged me to pay attention to what was going on in my life, but I kept ignoring them and overriding their messages. It took my body and my immune system collapsing, for me to finally start paying attention.

Bed ridden and unable to do anything other than sleep for weeks, provided me with the opportunity to 'wake up'.

As my entire life ground to a halt, I had no choice other than to listen to my intuition and connect with my inner guidance.

As you can imagine, after hitting this low point in my life I was ready to listen. I realised that my resistance was futile. I could no longer run from my internal pain and conflict. I became motivated to address and heal it, in a way that I hadn't been able to do before.

**Breaking free of self sabotage.**

Breaking free of self sabotage is to release your self from the thoughts, feelings, beliefs and actions that are interfering with your ability to achieve your weight loss goals.

When you free yourself from your own inner struggle in this way, you allow things to manifest much more easily. You will naturally change old beliefs and habits so that you can experience transformation and personal growth, along with increased levels of self awareness.

If you are experiencing self-sabotage it is important not to go into frustration, blame or apathy. It is far more powerful to enter the mode of the 'silent witness' and just observe what needs to be healed.

Many women tell me that they experience self sabotage when they would like to do good things for themselves, but for whatever reason are unable to do so. Often they tell me that they procrastinate on things, eat things they don't really want to eat or start binge eating as soon as they get close to realising their weight loss goals.

When you understand that self sabotage is the manifestation of your unconscious beliefs seeking your attention, then you can start to work with them. Awareness is always the first step in healing any inner conflict and sabotage.

# Create supportive beliefs.

*"People often become what they believe themselves to be. If I believe I cannot do something, it makes me incapable of doing it. But when I believe I can, then I acquire the ability to do it even if I didn't have it in the beginning."*

*~ Mahatma Gandhi*

Once you have questioned and cleared your old limiting weight loss beliefs, you can then enter the creative phase of reimagining what it is that you really want to create with your life. It is essential that whenever you clear an old limiting belief, that you replace it with something that is more fully in alignment with who you are becoming.

Nature abhors a vacuum. If you pull out a weed in your garden but don't replace it with the plants or flowers that you desire, another weed will swiftly grow back again to take its place.

It is the same with your beliefs. Once you have released and let go of a limiting weight loss belief, take the opportunity to create a new and exciting belief to replace it with.

### How do I create new weight loss beliefs?

Creating new weight loss beliefs, that support your health and wellbeing, is something that you must do for yourself. It is totally an inside job, one which nobody else can do it for you.

Creating new beliefs begins with your thoughts. As you upgrade your thoughts, your feelings and emotions will naturally change too. This, in turn, positively impacts upon your beliefs and future expectations.

The best place to start creating new weight loss beliefs is by activating your imagination. If you are wondering how you might be able to do this, take some time out to observe small children or make space for your own inner child to come out and play in your life.

Children are the masters of imagination. They have an unlimited sense of what is possible and are not encumbered by the same societal rules or constraints that most adults feel bound by. They learn best through their heightened sense of curiosity, experimentation, wonder and play.

Most children tend not to accept things on face value and have an almost obsessive infatuation with the question, 'But why?'

Creative thinking and dreaming are fundamental in the process of recreating your life. By actively using your imagination you immediately start to broaden your prospects and reshape your beliefs.

Take some time to ponder how you would like to transform your body, health, well being and life.

What kind of energy levels would you like to enjoy? What new forms of exercise might you like to try? What types of clothes would you like to wear? What childhood dreams would you like to realise?

Now think about what types of supportive weight loss thoughts and beliefs you would need to have in order to manifest your dreams into reality. As soon as something comes to mind be sure to write it down.

The table below provides a sample list of 'limiting beliefs' that can be replaced by 'supportive beliefs'.

| Limiting Beliefs | Supportive Beliefs |
|---|---|
| 'Losing weight is hard.' | 'Losing weight is easy when you know how.' |
| 'I will always be fat.' | 'I am becoming lighter every day.' |
| 'Weight problems run in my family.' | 'I am responsible for my own health and wellbeing.' |
| 'Food is my worst enemy. | 'Nourishing food nurtures my body, mind and soul.' |
| 'I hate exercising.' | 'I enjoy the freedom of moving my body.' |
| 'My family and friends don't support me.' | 'I surround myself with people who support me.' |
| 'My loved ones don't want me to change.' | 'I choose to be an inspiration for my loved ones.' |

| | |
|---|---|
| 'I hate my body.' | 'I am learning to love my body.' |
| 'Looking at food makes me gain weight.' | 'I choose to make healthy food choices.' |
| 'I am too old to lose weight.' | 'I am the perfect age to start listening to my body.' |
| 'My body feels like a prison.' | 'My body is my temple.' |

**Shift your beliefs and you will shift your world.**

Remember that everything inside you can change. When your internal world shifts, so too will your external world.

If you decide to upgrade an old belief such as 'eating healthy food is boring' to 'eating healthy food is fun' notice how quickly the world around you changes. As you change, so too does everything else in your life.

When you shift your beliefs in this way, what you are effectively doing is transforming the frequency of your consciousness. As you release your limiting beliefs and take on new supportive beliefs, without doing anything else at all, your mind will start to pay attention to a completely different set of phenomena.

Be on the lookout for uncanny synchronicities that begin to unfold in your life as a result of upgrading your beliefs. Through the shift in your belief, you will start to observe, notice and attract a very different life experience; one which allows 'healthy food' and 'fun' to be intimately linked together.

Don't be surprised if you start looking at things already present in your life in a completely different way.

You may start to notice healthy food everywhere. You might see cooking classes or workshops that you feel inclined to attend. You may notice healthy food or restaurants in your area that you had never seen before. Inspiring cookbooks may be 'given' to you. You may even experience chance meetings with like-minded people who also believe that 'healthy food' and 'fun' are possible. All of these things can support you on your weight loss healing journey.

What is so powerful about working with your beliefs in this way is that nothing else in your life needs to change, except for the quality of your thoughts. As you begin to think new thoughts and create new beliefs, you will literally create a whole new world for yourself.

Equipped with new supportive beliefs, you will be much better able to lose weight naturally, enrich your life experience and live more fully in alignment with your hopes, dreams and higher purpose.

## Reinforce supportive beliefs.

*"A belief is not merely an idea the mind possesses; it is an idea that possesses the mind."*

*~ Robert Oxton Bolt*

Once you have created your new supportive weight loss belief, it is essential that you reinforce the belief so that it becomes deeply embedded in your consciousness and natural way of being.

To reinforce your supportive weight loss belief you need to do 3 things.

1. Gather evidence to support your new belief.
2. Become passionate about your new belief.
3. Use repetition of thought to embed your new belief.

**1. Gather evidence to support your new weight loss belief.**

Reinforcing new supportive weight loss beliefs begins with being able to substantiate the belief with evidence and proof of your ability to lose weight naturally.

When I run workshops, I often spend time helping people identify and transform their limiting beliefs. To demonstrate how easy this can be, I invite participants to think of each of their beliefs as a table top.

Now for your typical table to stand strong, it requires four legs. If you take away one of those legs, the table will instantly become shaky and unstable. If you remove a second leg the table will probably wobble and collapse.

This is how it is with beliefs. For a belief to be strong, it needs 'support'. This support comes in the form of evidence that you take as true. This evidence can come in many different forms; from a 'truth' accepted in childhood, to something that you are sure about; to something you believe to be true from things you have read, to an opinion of someone you trust.

As soon as you remove the support (by creating doubt about the validity of a belief), it becomes shaky and unstable. If you can create enough doubt about an old belief then it will shatter, ready to be replaced and upgraded with a new and more empowering belief.

Now when you are reinforcing a new belief, you want to begin with the new supportive belief that you want to reinforce. Next you want to find overwhelming pieces of evidence to substantiate this new belief so that the mind begins to accept it as true.

I recommend that you start by finding at least 4 solid examples of evidence of why your new belief could become 'true for you' so that it can support you in becoming the person you are in the process of becoming.

## 2. Become passionate about your new weight loss belief.

Your new supportive weight loss beliefs will start to have real power when you can ignite them with energy, excitement and passion.

A powerful way to do this is to fully engage the imagination, including your 5 senses. This uses your sensory capabilities, which is the primary language that your body understands.

Start out by imagining how your new supportive weight loss belief will affect the course and destiny of your life. Notice what sensations and emotions naturally start to occur inside of you as you do this.

To amplify this process, you can also try actively engaging your five senses of sight (visual), sound (auditory), touch (kinesthetic), taste (gustatory) and smell (olfactory).

**Visualise:** How will your life look with your new belief? What types of clothes will you be wearing?

**Listen:** What music will you listen to? What will you say to yourself? What will other people say to you?

**Feel:** How will you feel about your life with your new belief? Will you feel happier? Healthier? More self confident? More energised? More aliveness?

**Taste:** How will your life taste with your new belief? What delicious and healthy new foods will you eat? What new recipes will you experiment with?

**Smell:** How will your life smell with your new belief? Does life smell fresher? What does your fresh food smell like?

It is okay if you don't get a response for all 5 senses; most people have different sensory preferences. Just focus on the ones that are strongest for you.

The key to reinforcing your new beliefs with this process is to see what emotions awaken within you. This is especially powerful when you begin to engage your imagination, along with your five senses and your passion.

### 3. Repeat your thoughts to embed your new belief.

Repeating a new supportive weight loss belief in your mind with great emotion is a sure fire way to transform it into something that has the power to inspire a completely new way of being. When you do this you are creating new neural pathways in your mind. The deeper the neural pathway created by your belief, the increased likeliness that it will positively influence your thoughts, behaviours and results in the future.

Creating supportive neural pathways are especially helpful when developing new lifestyle habits around healthy eating, drinking, exercising and sleeping. This process of repetition will at first be a conscious act, but very soon it will become unconsciously embedded within your cells that you will barely have to think about it.

Think back to when you first started to learn how to drive a car. Remember having to consciously think about changing gears, using the brakes, looking at your mirrors, indicating and steering, whilst also trying to keep an eye on the traffic around you as well? I am sure this will have felt quite awkward for you at first, but through practice and repetition, driving becomes second nature.

The process of reinforcing your new weight loss beliefs is similar. Begin by gathering as much evidence as you can find, to support the possibility and truth of your new weight loss beliefs.

The next thing to do is to allow yourself to become excited about your new life.

Think about what new possibilities could start to open up for you as you consciously and passionately redesign your life from the inside out.

To reinforce your new beliefs repeat this process frequently throughout your day. Allow new ideas and inspirations to emerge and motivate you on your journey to easily achieve your personal weight loss and healing goals.

## Boost your self-esteem.

*"Self confidence is the first requisite to great undertakings."*

*~ Dr. Samuel Johnson*

Self esteem is a term in psychology that is used to reflect a person's overall evaluation or appraisal of their personal worth. A positive relationship to the self is referred to as 'high self esteem' whereas a negative relationship to self is referred to as 'low self esteem'.

Many women get caught up in the yo-yo dieting trap and as a result suffer from damaged or very low self esteem. I know I certainly did. After a number of failed dieting attempts I had begun to lose faith in my ability to lose weight and in myself. So much so that it was negatively impacting other areas of my life. I blamed myself for my dieting failures and thought that I must be the one at fault.

I later discovered that low self esteem is a common experience for women of all shapes and sizes who have been caught up in the dieting trap.  The sad thing is that women are far more inclined to blame themselves rather than the dieting industry.

## Low self esteem = high profits.

The dieting industry is well aware of the correlation between low self esteem and high profits.  Women with low self esteem are far more likely to diet (even when they are not overweight) than women with high self esteem.

To achieve this, the dieting industry has carefully constructed a mirage of what a perfect woman's body should look like.  This leaves most normal women feeling totally inadequate, as if they do not 'measure up' or 'fall short' in some way.  Typically, this type of comparison results in low esteem and feelings of 'not being good enough.'

This kind of behaviour can have a devastating impact on how women feel about themselves.

What is less widely known is that the glossy pictures in celebrity magazines are almost always touched up and airbrushed to unattainable standards, using photo editing software.

In 2000, the UK magazine called 'Bliss' asked 2000 girls aged between the ages of 10 and 19 years old, how they felt about their bodies.  Nine out of ten confessed they weren't happy with how they looked and while only 19% of them were overweight, two thirds of them thought that they needed to lose weight.

## Self punishment creates low self esteem.

Dieting is a common way women unconsciously punish themselves in their lives.  It has the unintended result of placing self imposed deprivation, restriction and limitation on your life.  Unconsciously, when you suffer from low self esteem, you hold yourself back from living life on your own terms, with little regard for your personal dreams or goals.

The vicious dieting cycle is a perfect method for inflicting self punishment and pain.

If you are someone who regularly suffers from low self esteem and routinely places limitation on yourself, then realise that you are now being called to pay attention to that quiet, still voice within.

## The classic effects of low self esteem.

When I met Susan two years ago, she was experiencing the classic symptoms and effects of low self esteem.  She was in her early 30s, and she told me that she felt around 20lbs overweight, physically run down and totally uninspired about her life.

Although she had beautiful facial features, she kept them carefully concealed behind the thick glasses that she wore.  To the outside world she presented a sunny and cheerful disposition, but in her internal world she was beginning to feel incredibly unhappy.

In her breakthrough healing session, she revealed that her days were filled with a lingering pessimism and that she was having increasingly negative thoughts about herself and her life.

Whilst Susan liked her job, she was extremely tired from it.  She felt that it was 'draining her life force energy'.  She told me that she felt stuck and that she was secretly hoping that she might find some kind of way to feel different about herself.

I asked Susan what would need to happen, so that she could begin to move in the direction of what she truly desired.  From nowhere, out popped the words, *'I would have to leave my job.'*  We looked at each other in surprise.  Then she quickly added, *'I couldn't do that - my boss would kill me.'*

During our remaining time together, we addressed her feelings of fear and self-doubt.  Deep down she knew that there was a part of her that felt powerful and courageous and she wanted to reconnect with it again.  Through the session I could see her sense of self-confidence begin to return.  She left my healing room a woman ready to reclaim her joy for living.

When Susan returned to work a week or so later, she told her boss that she had decided to leave her job.  Her boss begged her to stay and promised to do everything she could to keep her.  True to her word, she managed to negotiate 3 months paid leave, as well as the promise of a new job on her return back to work.  As soon as she started her new role she fell in love with it and it was a perfect match for her skills and interests.

When I caught up with Susan recently, I got to witness first-hand, the personal transformation that she had undergone since our session. She looked very happy and exuded a healthy and radiant glow. She had lost her excess weight and was wearing figure hugging clothes, as well as a sexy new pair of glasses.

Susan shared all the amazing things that had happened to her after our breakthrough healing session. She noticed that she was able to address all the things that had been depleting her of energy and instead focus her energy on doing things which boosted her self esteem. She said that the healing work that we had done had totally shifted the way she felt about herself. This internal shift gave her the confidence she needed to be able to honestly express her true feelings to herself and to others.

She remarked that the excess weight that she had been carrying had naturally fallen off, as soon as she started to follow her personal path. Today she is enjoying living life on her own terms, in a way that is deeply honouring of all the different parts of herself and her personal needs.

**Low self esteem is an indication of unfulfilled potential.**

The areas in your life that you exhibit low self esteem are the ones where you are not realising your full potential.

Know that the process of healing self esteem happens naturally when you begin to take a holistic approach to your weight loss healing journey. Doing so creates more space in your life to discover new and supportive ways to address the real issues residing underneath your weight problems.

Being overweight is a powerful sign that life is calling you to grow beyond who you are being today. It is inviting you to step bravely and powerfully into your potential. From here you can connect with your untapped greatness. Consider that life is tapping you on the shoulder and asking you to display more of who you really are.

The biggest resources that you have in your life are your time and your energy, so you must learn how to use them wisely.

Spend your time and energy doing things that you enjoy and you will begin to feel better about yourself. This will result in a feeling of improved self confidence and put you firmly on your path to healing low self esteem and living an exciting life you love.

**Surround yourself with people that inspire you.**

If you are suffering with low self esteem, it is necessary to know that the people whom you surround yourself with, have the ability to strongly affect your self esteem.

Become aware of the power and influence that your family, friends and work colleagues can have on you. Whether consciously or unconsciously, they can influence the way you think, how you feel and what you do.

Surrounding yourself with positive and uplifting people is the little-but-powerful secret that you can use to begin building your self esteem levels. Spend as much time with people who believe in you and inspire you to be successful.

These people can help guide you on your path. You can connect with them by reading their books, listening to their audios or attending their workshops and retreats.

When other people believe in you, it becomes so much easier to believe in yourself.


**Creating the right support team.**

Building a support team will make your healing journey more enjoyable for you.

My naturopath was an incredible support person for me as I started on my healing journey towards reclaiming my health and wellbeing.

In addition, my parents and my aunt helped me to navigate my way through the many different natural approaches that were available. They helped me to find the right information so that I could naturally reclaim back my health and my body.

When I hit the bumps in the road, as inevitably you will too, it was my support team who were there to pick up the pieces.

They believed in me and my ability to succeed on my path. As well as their physical help, having their emotional support helped me to stay focused on the healing results that I wanted to achieve.

Having people around you, who can cheer you along on your journey, is going to be an important part of your success.

Your support team may come in the form of your family members, friends, health professionals, mentors, coaches or support groups.

Creating the right support team will make you stronger and help keep you committed to your healing path.

# PHASE 3:

# Heal Your Emotions

# Chapter Six – Emotional Eating

*"Weight loss is not just what you put on your plate, but also what happens to you in your life and how you respond to it. "*

*~ Katrina Love Senn, 2011*

| The Dieting Approach to Emotional Eating | The Healing Approach to Emotional Eating |
|---|---|
| ✘ Emotions must be controlled | ✓ Emotions want to be expressed |
| ✘ The problem is with the dieter | ✓ The problem is with the diet model |
| ✘ Driven by fear, guilt and obligation | ✓ Guided to courageously heal from within |
| ✘ Your emotions are dishonoured | ✓ Your emotions are deeply honoured |
| ✘ Uses a band aid approach | ✓ Addresses and heals the root cause |

## What is emotional eating?

*"Gluttony is an emotional escape, a sign something is eating us."*

*~ Peter De Vries.*

If you have tried everything to lose weight without success (particularly using the old model of dieting), then the time has come to explore how you use food to deal with your emotions.

Emotional eating is when food is used to manage, regulate and even medicate uncomfortable feelings on a regular or habitual basis. It can be used as a means to bury emotions or feelings that you don't want to feel or express.

Eating in this way is a very common 'coping strategy' used by women, of all shapes and sizes, to deal with every day stress, challenging situations or their life circumstances.

**Symptoms of emotional eating are wide and varied but can include:**

- Eating when you feel nervous, anxious or stressed.
- Eating when you feel sad, upset or lonely.
- Eating food to feel better or different.
- Eating food past the point of feeling full.
- Eating food too quickly.
- Eating food when you are bored or tired.
- Eating food with low levels of awareness.
- After eating food feeling filled with guilt, disgust or self hatred.
- After eating, feeling ashamed or embarrassed over the quantity or type of food consumed.

**I was an emotional eater.**

Being an emotionally sensitive person, whenever I experienced feeling rejected, stressed or hurt I would use food as a way to make myself temporarily feel better. This worked, for a while. After years of living my life in this way I began to gain weight. I tried to lose weight by dieting, which only led me to struggle even more with my weight and confidence. This led me to focus exclusively on what I was eating, instead of examining the inner world of my thoughts and emotions.

Looking back, I can see how I used dieting as a way to relentlessly punish myself. I imposed strict rules around my food; counting, controlling and measuring it. I used food to manipulate, suppress, numb, push down and avoid my fear based feelings of frustration, rejection, fear, loneliness, anger and sadness.

What I didn't realise was that by eating emotionally, I was disconnecting from my true feelings and instead distracting myself with food. Eating was a way to soothe the pain of the emotions that I wasn't ready to deal with. It had the benefit of temporarily masking my pain and it made me feel good again.

For many years, I was unconscious and unaware of my destructive eating patterns. I thought that this was how I was supposed to lose weight. It was these specific patterns that kept me feeling frustrated with my weight and myself. With the benefit of hindsight, I can see now why I struggled to lose weight for so long.

As soon as I stopped focusing all of my energy on food and started to focus on my feelings, I was able to turn everything around. I learnt how to ditch my dieting approach and instead open to a completely new paradigm with a fresh appreciation and understanding of weight loss.

I started to look within and began learning how to express my true feelings to myself and others. As I did this, I began to feel better. I gained more confidence and as a result, began to lose weight naturally.

It seems I was not alone in my struggle with emotional eating. Well known celebrities like Kate Winslet, Kristie Alley, Christina Aguilera, Jessica Simpson and Janet Jackson have spoken openly and honestly about their personal issues with emotional eating.

**Why diets don't work for emotional eaters.**

Dieting does not work because it only serves as a band aid approach to emotional eating. Diets only serve to mask the symptoms of the real problem. They do not address or heal the root cause of the situation. When you don't address the root cause, the problem will keep repeating itself until it is healed, much in the same way a weed will keep growing back unless pulled out from the roots.

Most emotional eaters know a lot about food and nutrition. They've often read a number of 'diet' books. They know what foods to eat, but yet, they still struggle to lose weight.

Dieting creates a feeling of restriction, starvation and deprivation. Trying to stop eating certain foods is futile if done without addressing the underlying emotional issues. Dieting does not deal with the problem at the root cause. It is only a short term solution that will typically leave you feeling worse.

**Emotional eating is a sign of emotional hunger.**

When you are eating emotionally you aren't eating because you are 'physically hungry' but because you are 'emotionally hungry'.

'Emotional hunger' feels very different from 'physical hunger'. In fact, if you are an emotional eater it is entirely possible that you may have even forgotten what real physical hunger feels like at all.

'Physical hunger' craves real, whole foods and proper nutrition. After eating real food, your body will feel nourished and satiated and will only require food when it becomes physically hungry again.

'Emotional hunger' on the other hand typically craves junk and processed foods. When you are feeling emotionally hungry, no matter what you eat, it will not satisfy you.

When you are emotionally hungry, even after consuming large quantities of food, it is also entirely possible to still feel 'empty'. Eating when you are emotionally hungry is like trying to fill a bottomless void. No matter what you eat, it can never be filled with food.

Emotional cravings can come on fast and seemingly from nowhere. The hunger pangs always begin with your feelings and not your stomach. With unconscious repetition, emotional eating can very quickly become your default style of dealing with stress. When you use this eating approach as your emotional 'coping strategy', all you are really doing is creating a fleeting distraction to avoid having to deal with your true feelings.

Next time you experience food cravings, ask yourself 'where do I feel hungry?' Distinguish if the hunger you feel is from your stomach or your emotions. If the hunger is coming from your emotions, keep in mind that no amount of food will ever be able to fill or satiate it.

## Stop feeding emotional hunger with fake foods.

Fake foods are typically laden with chemical stimulants that are designed to affect your brain chemistry and heighten your desire for even more junk food. Immediately after eating this type of food, your body and brain are stimulated. Energy levels go up but then they crash very quickly too.

The real problem with emotional eating is that the internal change is always a temporary one. Although food has the ability to squash down your uncomfortable feelings, they can quickly resurface again.

As soon as the good feeling, derived from the food, has disappeared from your mouth, you will be left with your original pain, along with additional feelings of anger, frustration, disgust or shame.

You may feel that the only thing you can do to stop that feeling from coming back is to eat more. While this may be tempting, this is definitely not the path to creating a vibrantly healthy and emotionally fulfilling life.

## Using food to feel better.

Emotional eating can become a problem when you routinely use food as a way to feel better about yourself and your life. 'Binge eaters' typically use food to escape situations that are too painful to deal with or that they just don't know how to deal with.

Jen was a client that I worked with from the UK. She was 44 years of age and told me that she had never known love.

As a child she was handed from one adoption agency to the next. She grew up with no sense of belonging and as an adult still carried the pain of rejection, sadness and disappointment. She was smart and witty, with a smile that could light up any room, but on the inside she hid her innermost feelings of shame and not being good enough. She hated herself and suffered low self-esteem. She felt inadequate and deeply embarrassed about herself and her life. From years of hunching over and hiding herself, she had developed bad posture with rounded shoulders. She dressed in big, black, baggy clothing to hide her body.

Jen's drug of choice was chocolate. She had come to learn that chocolate was the only thing that she could count upon. Chocolate was her solace from the cruel world she had been born into. Jen knew that chocolate would be waiting for her the moment she stepped through her front door each night after work. Eating chocolate had the ability to make Jen temporarily feel much better about herself. But eating so much chocolate over the years, had taken a heavy toll on her physical body.

During our break-through healing session, Jen was able to see that she was seeking more than chocolate. What she was truly seeking was love and support. It was like a light went on in her life. She had an 'a-ha' moment. She realised that she would binge eat whenever she felt unloved or not worthy of love.

She began to understand that food was there to fuel and nourish her body, not to provide a substitute for the love that she craved. With this awareness Jen was able to focus upon creating relationships that gave her the sense of connection, love and friendship that she had been previously searching for in chocolate.

Jen left my clinic room with the awareness that her past was not her future. Yes, she had lived through a challenging upbringing, but this was not who she was.

Jen realised that her past was her past. She made a decision to leave it behind her and instead focus her energy on tapping into the possibilities of today.

With this new attitude and awakened spirit of curiosity she began to wonder what kind of tomorrows she would be creating. Although tentative at the beginning, by the end of our break-through healing session she was a woman who was aware that she was deserving and worthy of love.

She told me that she wanted to begin nurturing herself with food. She felt excited to begin pursuing other activities to continue healing the mental, emotional and spiritual aspects of her life as well.

**Our bodies are adaptable.**

Our bodies are very adaptable, so occasional emotional eating is not going to cause you long term harm. Where it becomes problematic is when you routinely use it as a way to feel better about life.

The challenge of using emotional eating as a coping strategy, is that it only ever deals with the surface level concern and not the emotional cause. If emotional eating or self sabotage is an ongoing problem for you, then addressing the root cause has the potential to transform everything for you. We explore the emotional root cause later in this chapter.

Emotional eating can only ever provide temporary relief. With time you will require increasingly larger quantities of food to numb your emotional pain and anguish.

Pay attention to your feelings as they hold the key to your emotional healing.

**Food addictions, illness and disease.**

Chronic emotional eating can manifest in out-of-control eating behaviours, such as food binges, purging and food addictions. This in turn can lead to weight gain, obesity and a whole host of other chronic, degenerative diseases.

The thing that can make food addictions much more challenging to deal with than other forms of addiction, is that you still need to eat. With drug or alcohol addictions for example, you can always go 'cold turkey' when you move into a recovery phase.

Eating food is essential to life. To overcome your food addictions you must do so by continuing to eat. To do this effectively you need to learn healthy ways to manage and express your feelings without using food.

Becoming conscious of how you feel can help you to break the cycle of emotional eating. As you listen to your inner voice, you can learn how to treat yourself with respect and love. As you tune in to your feelings and emotions, your relationship to food and your eating patterns will begin to shift naturally.

Losing weight for good is about addressing your emotions so that you can break free of your food addictions. In doing so, you will create a sense of freedom and joy around food and in your life.

---

# Exercise: Understanding emotional eating.

Next time you eat emotionally, ask yourself the following questions:

1. What feelings am I trying to dull or numb out?

   ..........................................................................

2. How can I safely connect with and honour my feelings?

   ..........................................................................

3. What am I hiding from myself or others?

   ..........................................................................

# Emotional Eating Quiz.

Are you an emotional eater? Circle your answers and then count up your yes responses. Use the interpretation below to find out the role emotional eating plays in your life.

**Food and feelings.**

| | |
|---|---|
| Do you find that eating or buying food helps you to feel better? | YES/NO |
| Do you feel emotionally different after you eat? | YES/NO |
| Does eating help you ease stress or discomfort? | YES/NO |

**Food and control.**

| | |
|---|---|
| Do you often feel out of control around food? | YES/NO |
| Do you feel that your eating is out of control? | YES/NO |

**Food and emotions.**

| | |
|---|---|
| Do you often eat when you are not hungry? | YES/NO |
| Do you eat or crave fake foods? | YES/NO |

**Food and rewards.**

| | |
|---|---|
| Do you eat food for pleasure? | YES/NO |
| Do you regularly reward yourself with food? | YES/NO |

**Food and guilt.**

| | |
|---|---|
| Do you other people watching you eat? | YES/NO |
| After eating do you feel guilty or ashamed? | YES/NO |
| Do you ever eat in private? | YES/NO |

**Now add up how many YES you marked.**

**Interpretation of your score:**

0-1     It is unlikely that your emotional eating is harmful for you.

2-3     You engage in some emotional eating but it's unlikely to be harmful.

4-9     Emotional eating may be a moderate challenge for you. Emotional healing can help.

10-12     Emotional eating is a challenge for you. Use emotional healing to help resolve this.

## The 3 layers of emotion.

*"Tenderness and kindness are not signs of weakness and despair but manifestations of strength and resolution."*

*~ Kahlil Gibran*

One area that most traditional weight loss approaches overlook is the power of your emotions to influence your food choices, life decisions and state of being.

Your emotions are powerful and can significantly impact all areas of your life, including your health, wellness and even your ability to lose weight.

Everyone eats emotionally from time to time. Given the intricate role food plays in our everyday lives, it's an inevitable part of being human.

Where emotional eating becomes problematic, is when it moves from being an occasional occurrence, to your default style of eating. This happens when your emotions become the main driver of when, how and what you eat.

If you can relate to this, then the time has come to take a closer look at the impact your inner world of emotions is having upon your food choices as well as your weight.

## Advertisers understand the power of emotions.

Advertisers understand the power of human emotions and the influence they have upon the decision-making process. This is why they create multi-million dollar advertising campaigns designed specifically to trigger different aspects of your emotions and psyche.

Advertisers know that they can by-pass your rational decision making process by activating your emotional brain. Through doing this they know that they can influence you to make emotionally charged, impulse buying decisions instead of carefully considered, rational ones. These techniques are particularly used by the food industry to stimulate you into buying fake foods.

## The 3 layers of emotion.

Each emotion you experience carries an energetic frequency. Some emotions are dark and heavy and create 'dis-ease' within your body. Others are light and flowing, bringing you feelings of health, happiness and wellbeing.

To understand the role emotions play in weight gain, it is first necessary to understand the 3 primary 'layers of emotion' that we experience as human beings. These 3 layers of emotion are:

- Layer 1: Fear based emotions
- Layer 2: Courage based emotions
- Layer 3: Love based emotions

Let's take a closer look at these different layers individually.

# The 3 Layers of Emotion

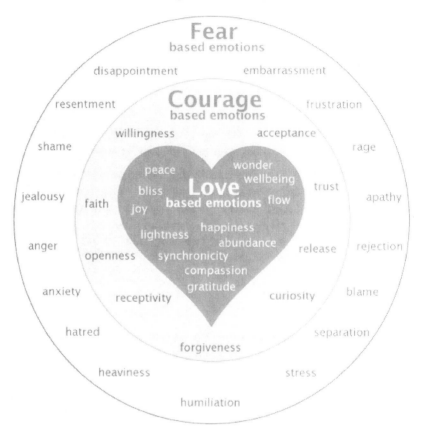

**Layer 1: Fear based emotions.**

Fear based emotions are the emotions that are largely responsible for weight gain in women.

These emotions are heavy in nature and are usually the result of some kind of perceived threat, whether real or imagined. Whenever you experience a fear based emotion that you don't process or let go of, you hold it within the cellular memories of your body. The emotion gets held here until you release and heal it. It is likely that many of your old fear based emotions come from your childhood, at a time when you didn't have the emotional resources or maturity to deal with them appropriately.

The storage of these fear based emotions can initially go unnoticed physically, but as they start to accumulate they can manifest as excess weight within the body.

Many women unknowingly make their way through life carrying around a 'metaphysical backpack' of fear based emotions. This backpack gets progressively heavier as it fills with a life time of unaddressed fear based experiences.

From time to time these old fears will come up in the body for healing and release. These feelings can be uncomfortable. As a result many women override these feelings with food, rather than dealing with them directly.

Using food to squash fear based emotions in this way can certainly have a short term pay off. However, if the emotions are left unaddressed, they can cause chronic disturbance and disharmony within your body, mind and spirit.

Some examples of fear based emotions include: frustration, shame, embarrassment, humiliation, disgust, rejection, hatred, anger, rage, jealousy, revenge, boredom, stress, anxiety, pessimism, impatience, overwhelm, disappointment, doubt, worry, blame, discouragement, revenge, jealousy, insecurity, guilt, fear, grief, depression, despair, powerlessness, hopelessness, unworthiness, helplessness, indifference and self pity.

**Layer 2: Courage based emotions.**

The second layer of emotion is called 'courage based emotions'.

True courage is the ability to confront fear based emotions. With regards to emotional eating, this means having a willingness to turn your gaze inwards and start addressing the emotional fears and challenges of your life, as well as your relationship with food.

Without this willingness, you will remain a victim of circumstance, living out the default patterns of your habits, programming, conditioning and past experiences.

Courage based emotions open the doorway to your growth, healing and health. It is from this place that long term sustainable weight loss starts to become a very real possibility.

Using our 'backpack metaphor', having courage means being willing to unzip the backpack and take a close look at the emotions that you have been consciously or unconsciously carrying around with you. By doing this you may instantly see things that you no longer need and can let go of immediately. Other old fear based emotions may require a longer process of healing and release work.

When you begin to realise that you don't have to carry all these fear based emotions with you, you will immediately feel lighter. This act begins to set you free by releasing you from the shackles of your past.

As you live from your courage based emotions, you effectively begin to move beyond your fears as well as your comfort zone. By doing this you open your life to excitement, growth and deep healing.

Courage is the pathway to self confidence and living more fully connected to your dreams. As you immerse yourself in this process, you may begin to feel bolder, more creative and more adventurous.

You may even start considering doing things that you would never normally do or have always longed to do but felt you lacked the courage. As you do, invite in the new experiences. Give yourself permission to become more of who you really are and express the 'real' you.

These are all positive signs that you are living more courageously. As you continue to do this, you will discover the resources necessary to keep moving your life forward in the direction of your dreams and what you truly value.

Some examples of courage based emotions include: willingness, acceptance, receptivity, trust, faith, forgiveness, curiosity, openness and bravery.

**Layer 3: Love based emotions.**

The third layer of emotion and the deepest part of your being is called 'Love based emotions'.

When you release fear based emotions and allow the energy of courage to infuse your body, mind and spirit, you will be more easily able to connect with the higher frequencies of Love based emotions.

The Love I am talking about here is not the romantic notion of love. It is the Love that exists at the very core and essence of your being. Everything melts in the presence of this Love.

It is the space from which all true, deep and lasting healing comes from. It is the space where you get to see the true gifts of your excess weight and realise that you no longer need it to teach you. When we strip ourselves bare, Love is all that we are. Our fears merely cover over what has always been there.

Love based emotions enable you to live more fully in alignment with your higher self and authentic truth, so that you can do more of the things that you want with your life. Being in this heart centred space will connect your mind, body and spirit to feelings of inner peace and joy.

Living with Love is a way to live in truth with your life purpose and spiritual path. When you live from a place of love, gratitude and compassion your life works on all levels. You realise that within you is all the confidence you need to live in a self-directed way. From this place you get to realise that you are the Love that you have been looking for all along.

Some examples of Love based emotions include: happiness, lightness, gratitude, abundance, bliss, joy, compassion, synchronicity, flow, Love, peace, wonder and wellbeing.

## Emotional eating is a symptom.

*"Emotion always has its roots in the unconscious and manifests itself in the body."*

*~ Irene Claremont de Castillejo*

Many women, who eat emotionally, think that emotional eating is their problem. It isn't. Emotional eating is merely symptomatic of a deeper issue.

Regardless of what you hear on the latest infomercial, your emotional eating isn't a sign to go on a diet, pop a pill or have your stomach stapled. Your emotional eating is a call for emotional healing. It's a call to get real with yourself and to take back your power and your life.

Emotional eating is the scab or casing that lays on the surface of a deeper wound. It is an indicator that there is some healing work that needs to be done beneath the surface of the skin. Unfortunately, picking at the wound will never heal it.

**Exploring childhood patterns.**

When looking for an explanation of your behavioural patterns as an adult, it is often best to start tracing them back to emotional themes of your childhood.

The behaviours that won you attention, love and approval as a child, will often become your default strategies for getting attention, love, acceptance and approval as an adult.

Take a moment to think back to what 'role' you played as you were growing up. You can get a good idea by thinking about what other people said about you. This will give you an idea of how you learned how to get attention and thereby noticed within your family and social circles.

Were you the good girl who played by the rules? Were you the quiet or shy one? Or were you the loud, boisterous, rebellious or naughty girl?

Although this childhood strategy may have suited your individual situation perfectly as you were growing up, there is every possibility that it is no longer appropriate for you as an adult.

The trouble is that most of us are still operating from the same unconscious strategies that we used when we were young, even though they may be totally inappropriate or self defeating as an adult.

**Peeling back the layers.**

Now I want you to imagine that it is winter. It's cold and you are wearing a long winter jacket to keep yourself warm. You are so grateful for the jacket and you hate to think what your life would be like without it.

Now I want you to turn the clock forward in time and imagine that it is now summer. The weather is warm and sunny. You are still wearing the jacket but it is making you feel hot and bothered and as a result you are unsure about what to do.

Now there are many different ways you could deal with this feeling of being hot and bothered. Potentially you could:

- Complain about the problem to a friend.
- Talk through your problem with a therapist.
- Take medication to cool your body temperature.
- Move out of the sunshine and sit in the shade.

Now these different strategies may very well offer you some kind of temporary relief from your discomfort, but none of them offer you more than a 'band aid' solution to your suffering.

To bring about a long term solution there are two things you must do:

(1) Address the real problem (wearing a winter jacket in summer time); and
(2) Heal the problem (remove the winter jacket).

It seems pretty obvious really.

Now when it comes to emotional eating, I see many women live out this same seemingly ridiculous pattern. They look for a temporary band aid solution to their weight gain (diets, weight loss pills, lap bands, surgery) that don't address the real underlying emotional problem that created the weight gain in the first place.

**Using emotional eating as a default coping strategy.**

Several years ago, I worked with a lady who had a very troubled childhood. It was a very difficult time for her and years later she still held very strong childhood memories of the anger and violence that she grew accustomed to in her family home. Her parents fought on a regular basis and she had never done any inner work to address or heal these stressful childhood experiences.

As a child, the only coping strategy that provided her with any sense of comfort was eating. When she ate food she experienced a sense of safety and protection that she didn't otherwise receive at home. She described the feeling of eating as soothing, like 'being wrapped up in a warm fluffy blanket.'

As she grew older, eating food became her chosen way to relieve fear or anxiety. Food soothed her whenever she felt stressed or emotional. It was food that she used to receive the feelings of safety and security in a troublesome home environment that was lacking in both.

Now while this strategy provided her with the comfort she needed when she was a little girl, now a grown woman in her 40's, emotional eating had become her biggest problem.

When she was able to make the link between her emotional eating patterns and her unmet emotional needs, she was able to seek out healthier and more nourishing ways to nurture herself. As a result, her excess weight started to fall away naturally. Losing weight for her was a graceful process without dieting or struggle.

**Become aware of emotional triggers.**

To understand emotional eating more fully, it is important to appreciate that the act of emotional eating is a process. And that process begins with an emotional trigger.

An 'emotional trigger' is a thought or feeling that activates an unhealed emotional wound resulting in a particular behavioural response. For the emotional eater, that response may be an overwhelming desire to eat food, especially processed or junk food.

When you feel 'emotionally triggered', you may feel a fear based emotion such as anger, frustration or sadness well up inside of you. This experience may bring up unhealed emotions associated with past events in your life as well. For most women this triggering can be quite unconscious, particularly while it occurs in the moment.

Instead of being with this feeling and allowing it to come up naturally for exploration, expression or healing, you may consider it easier to just suppress the feeling by eating or drinking something. When you do this you are effectively using food to squash down or get rid of your uncomfortable fear based feelings.

To give you an illustration, imagine that you are at work and your boss says something that upsets you. This exchange may trigger a secret desire to leave your job and pursue something more fulfilling.

Given the fears you may also have about leaving your job, you may feel uncomfortable in expressing how you really feel about the situation and causing a confrontation. If you are an emotional eater, to cope with the tension created by this dilemma, you may choose to:

- Eat a chocolate bar or muffin to make yourself feel better.
- Go out for lunch but eat or drink too much.
- Go out for drinks after work to unwind.

Each one of these approaches, although possibly effective in removing the pain of the situation, will have done little to address the underlying problem – your desire to find more fulfilling work.

If this emotional eating strategy is repeated any time you experience seemingly un-resolvable tension at work or in other areas of your life, it is pretty easy to see how emotional eating can start to become a very real problem.

**You always have the power to choose.**

If you are an emotional eater and you have been triggered or are dealing with an 'un-resolvable' moment of tension, you have 2 basic behavioural choices you can make:

a)   To respond in fear; or
b)   To step into courage

If you respond in fear, you will more than likely default to the path of 'emotional eating' to appease your awkward and uncomfortable feelings.  If you choose to step into courage, you will be on the path to 'emotional healing'.  It really is a simple choice.  Either you can choose the path of emotional eating or emotional healing as shown below:

Emotional Triggers

Choice (a): Emotional Eating

Fear response → Emotional eating → Weight gain

Emotional trigger

Choice (b): Emotional Healing

Step into courage → Address the root cause → Heal with Love

In the next 2 sections we will explore these two choices in more detail.

## The path of emotional eating.

*"There seemed to be endless obstacles... it seemed that the root cause of them all was fear."*

*Joanna Field*

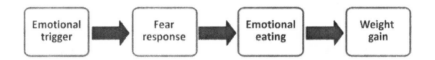

At the root of all emotional eating patterns is some kind of fear based emotional trigger that leads to a fear response. These fear based emotions lead to episodes of emotional eating and ultimately to weight gain.

For most emotional eaters, this path is chosen by default, largely because they unconsciously think that it is their only choice.

The path of emotional eating is illustrated in the flow diagram and discussed below. (We will explore the path of emotional healing in the next section of the book).

### 1. Fear response.

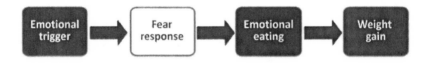

The fear response creates an energetic contraction that stops women from losing weight and moving forward in the direction of their dreams. It serves as a natural form of resistance that can keep you living small.

Fear keeps your heart and soul closed. Your body and mind become disconnected from each other as well. In the moment it can hold you back from really appreciating your true beauty and the innate greatness that exists at your core.

Based on my coaching, healing and teaching experience, it is fear that keeps women stuck. Living within the confines of fear, creates frustrating and unfulfilling lives and inhibits women from expressing who they really are and what is most important to them.

Fear is a powerful emotion. It can be very restrictive and controlling, keeping you wrapped up in old patterns. Fear can hold you back from living your true potential and prevent you from experiencing all the joy, love, magic and bliss that is freely available to you in your life.

Living with fear is in effect like living in a prison of your own making. Now even though living in this prison of fear can be challenging and stressful, it can have a comfortable familiarity to it. So much so, that many would prefer to stay within the confines of what they know rather than confront their fears and step into the unknown. This is a natural part of human nature, but it does not need to be your defining experience of life.

To leave this prison of fear, all you need to do is have the courage to open the door and walk through it.

You can always choose to be more adventurous and courageous. Rather than allowing fear to paralyse you, use it to drive, motivate and excite you into living a value-driven life filled with meaning and purpose.

Often women tell me things that they would absolutely love to do. When I ask them *"why don't you do it?"*, they often look at me in shock. One woman even said to me "Oh I could never do that."

Unfortunately, fear is the thief of many unlived dreams.

## 2. Emotional eating.

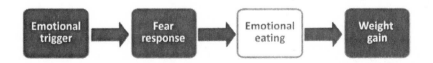

Once an emotional eater has been triggered, the discomfort of the fear response will often lead them to eat something.

Most emotional eaters will have what I call a favoured 'drug of choice', much in the same way that an alcoholic will have a favourite 'drink of choice'. Most emotional eaters will have a favourite chocolate bar, ice cream or biscuit which they use to dull their pain. Sandra's 'food of choice' was red wine and dark chocolate. Louise favoured milk chocolate with almonds and Lena's was anything sweet and sugary. Monica's food of choice was chocolate muffins.

Once conscious of their emotional crutches, when these food cravings hit they could make different choices for themselves. Awareness of your emotional cravings has the power to free you from the binds of food addictions.

Living fearfully keeps you small and can create the desire to 'swallow your feelings' rather than express them. Typically this happens when you choose to 'stuff down' uneasy feelings with food rather than express yourself.

If you've ever felt emotional and have been told to just get over it, move on, don't worry about it, forget about it or it doesn't matter, then you're not alone.

I used to swallow my feelings of anger and frustration to avoid upsetting other people. Even as a child I was a natural peace-keeper. I learnt that expressing my true feelings was neither appreciated nor appropriate. As a young child I learnt that it was best to keep quiet and be good.

Swallowing your feelings, doesn't mean that they will disappear or magically go away. If not expressed, these bottled feelings get held in your body. If you continue to ignore them, your life force energy can become stuck and stagnant. When your energy gets stuck, so too does your life.

Stuck energy creates an energetic disturbance and imbalance within your body. This can manifest in negative emotions and you may feel angry, lonely, upset, stressed, resentful hurt, disappointed, sad, spiteful, jealous, regretful, apathetic, fearful, anxious, depressed, frustrated or scared.

Other powerful indicators that your life force energy has become stuck include excess weight, lethargy, exhaustion and illness. In extreme cases, your body may even collapse or break down, just as mine did.

Emotional eating is calling you to sit up and pay attention to what isn't working in your life. Maybe something from your past is ready to transform. It could be that a painful memory, past trauma or life experience is ready to be released and healed, so that a natural flow can be restored to your life.

Emotional eating can be stopped when you have the courage to look within and start releasing both your conscious and unconscious fears.

## 3. Weight gain.

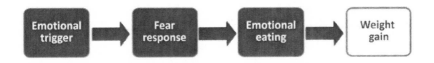

The fear based protection that you seek from emotional eating, will most likely result in weight gain, if left unaddressed.

When you live from a place of fear, your body requires barriers and layers of protection, just in case 'something bad happens'. The extra weight you are carrying may simply be your body's way of insulating you from the world and 'keeping you safe.'

When you look deep within yourself, you may be able to see and understand the real reason for carrying this protective layer. You may already know the reason or alternatively, you may need to spend a little time to find the unhealed pain that you have buried inside of you.

All of your unexpressed thoughts, emotions and feelings are stored physically in your body. The types of physical problems that you experience and even where your body fat is stored, can give you clues as to what emotions have been numbed out or suppressed.

Your suppressed feelings may be so old that you do not even remember where they originally came from. This is normal and to be expected. Healing emotional eating happens naturally, when 'old stuff' is gently expressed and released from your body and your life.

On my own journey, I carried a lot of my excess weight around my neck, throat and chest. When I was younger I had a hard time voicing my opinion and expressing my true feelings. I was afraid of being heard and especially of saying the wrong thing.

Energetically I used to store a lot of my repressed feelings in my throat. This not only resulted in excess weight gain in this area, but also contributed to the asthma and breathing problems I used to experience as well. Healing the feelings stored in this region of my body was a big part of my weight loss journey. As I gained confidence in my voice and expressing myself, my excess weight shifted naturally.

If you are overweight, know that your body hasn't made a mistake. All it is doing is giving you important information and feedback about how you are living your life.

Just know that it is possible to heal your old emotions by gently releasing them from your physical body, as well as your energy field. Always remember that it is your pain and you can work with it in any way that you choose. Only you will know when you are ready to actively start working with it.

The good news is that, the mere act of becoming conscious of your inner world begins the process of moving this stuck energy out of your body. As you move this old energy, you initiate the process of transformation and healing.

Looking back at your past and embarking upon your own inner healing work does take courage. You may decide that now isn't really the time for you to be doing this kind of work and that is okay. Within you, you will know when the time is right for you to do so.

Whether or not you choose to do your healing now, I congratulate you for being open hearted and willing to even just explore what it takes to heal. It's an amazing human accomplishment in and of itself.

**Addressing and releasing fear.**

A couple of years ago, I was working with a client at a retreat centre in the Greek Islands. She had been a school teacher for over 20 years and harboured a dream to change careers. In recent years, she had been on many courses learning new skills and had completed a Life Coaching qualification. While she dreamed of one day becoming a coach, there was a part of her that felt afraid.

She described her fear as 'paralysing.' So much so, that she confessed that she had been eating emotionally for years in order to combat her fear. She told me that she would binge eat chocolate at home and that she didn't know what she could do about it.

Her eating habits were a source of deep embarrassment and shame and she was desperate to regain control over her life.

As I began working with her, I asked to describe her fear, with as much vivid detail as possible. She replied that her fear made her feel as if she was on a diving board that was so high above the water that she couldn't even bear to walk down the diving board, let alone look down over the side.

In the session, we worked with the visual image and metaphor of the diving board, by reducing its' size and shape, as well as adding in other details such as lovely, crystal clear, glistening, warm water for her to jump into.

By the end of the session she was amazed that her fear had completely gone. She had transformed her fear and was now feeling excited about leaving her job to set up her new business!

Even though nothing had 'physically' changed in her life, her mental pictures had shifted, together with her emotional response. Finally, she felt as if she was ready to put her emotional eating behind her and move forward with her new career.

A few days after the session, she told me with great joy, that she felt free of her chocolate cravings too!

When your courage is bigger than your fear, you can break free. This doesn't mean that fear is not present, but rather that you have grown to a place where you are bigger than your fears.

When you choose to let go of fear and step into courage you really can live a magical and meaningful life. By doing so you are giving yourself permission to be who you really are.

## The path of emotional healing.

*"The struggle of life is one of our greatest blessings. It makes us patient, sensitive, and Godlike. It teaches us that although the world is full of suffering, it is also full of the overcoming of it."*

*~ Helen Keller*

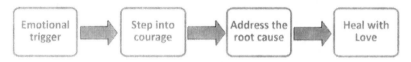

The path of emotional healing is a choice that is available to every emotional eater. However it is not a path that every emotional eater is aware of.

When you release fear and your old stuck emotions, you begin to activate your life force energy and your body's own self healing abilities. This in turn will naturally reduce the impulse to eat emotionally.

The best time to become present to the choice of emotional healing is when you have been emotionally triggered. Rather than defaulting into an emotional eating episode (as we explored in the last section), see it as a perfect opportunity to look deeply into what is really going on internally for you.

This process will help you to reconnect your body and mind, whilst also reducing your desire to eat emotionally.

In this section we will introduce some key principles of emotional healing. In the subsequent sections we will look at the individual components of emotional healing as illustrated in the flow diagram above.

## (1) Step into courage.

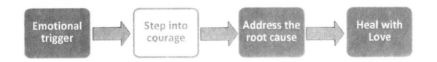

Your emotional eating is calling you to have the courage to look within and change something in your life. When you feel triggered and the desire to eat emotionally comes over you, you have a decision to make. You can either choose to:

     a)   Emotionally eat; or

     b)   Have the courage to heal the emotion.

Choosing to succumb to fear and eat, will keep you stuck in the cycle of emotional eating. Choosing to step into courage and work with the feeling will open you up to the path of emotional healing.


### Choosing courage over fear.

The Latin base of the word courage is 'cor', which means heart. To live with courage means to rise above your fears and follow the wisdom of your heart.

Choosing courage over fear will help you to overcome emotional eating. When you live with courage, permanent weight loss becomes possible. By facing your fears and healing your emotional pain, you will instantly change the relationship you have with food and yourself.

Courage gives you the ability to be receptive to new ideas, do things differently and go outside of what is normally comfortable for you. It also assists you to question the commonly held beliefs and behaviours of your family, friends and society as a whole, so that you can discover and walk your own path in life.

Stepping into courage gives you the ability to turn up the volume on your inner guidance, so that you can live more fully in alignment with your true values. As you progress you will find it becomes easier to trust yourself and your intuition. When you step into courage, doing what is right for you will become second nature.

Having the courage to explore your inner world will help you to heal your emotional eating. Below we explore four powerful ways where the quality of courage can help you on your weight loss healing journey.

- The courage to express yourself.
- The courage to be creative.
- The courage to be sensitive.
- The courage to go after your dreams.

**(a) The courage to express yourself.**

Expressing your true emotions is a great anti-dote to emotional eating. How many times have you gone to express something you were feeling only to have that feeling squashed down with food? Living a life filled with meaning and purpose starts with having the courage to express your true feelings.

Expressing who you really are may mean dedicating some time and space to reconnecting with yourself. Maybe your desire to live a more intuitive, creative and spiritual life has been buried inside of you for a long time as you navigated the 'real world' of education, career, money, relationships and family.

Begin by honestly expressing your feelings to yourself. Using a journal is an excellent way of doing this. When you are comfortable with this you may want to start sharing your feelings with other people. By honestly communicating your feelings to yourself and others, you can radically transform your life and help to heal your emotional eating. As you journal, ask yourself *'What emotion am I feeling?'*

Only when you express your true feelings to yourself and to others are you able to let go of them. As you let them go, you release the hold that they have on your life and allow emotional healing to take place.

**(b) The courage to be creative.**

Emotional eating and excess weight gain can often be signs of blocked creativity. Many women may not even know that they are creative. Having the courage to explore your creative and artistic self could be something that is incredibly healing for you.

For many years, I mistakenly thought that my sister got all the creative genes in our family. But with the benefit of hindsight, I can now see that my blocked creativity was a big contributing factor in my emotional eating. Today I have a deep connection to my inner artist and I love to nurture her with cooking, writing, travelling, teaching, painting and playing.

My break-through healing clients and yoga students often come to me curious about how best to unlock and express their creative talents.

Sarah Helena, a young lady from Sweden, had a profound break through during a yoga class that I was teaching in the Greek islands. During the class she got a strong intuitive message to start changing her habits and start honouring and loving her body. In the class she made a personal commitment to stop abusing her body and to start being kind to herself. She knew this would involve giving up smoking.

By looking after herself in this way she would be more fully able to honour her creative talents as a singer and musician. Afterwards she shared with me what had happened to her during the class. We talked about how her creative energy had likely been blocked by her old addictions. As soon as she released her old fear-based emotions, her creative energy was able to begin moving freely again.

What untapped creative potential resides in you, just waiting to be expressed? If you have not yet had a chance to fully explore your true creative potential, know that this could be the perfect time to begin.

When you feed and nourish your creativity you will begin to feel alive. The power of your life force energy will once again begin to pulse through your veins, filling you with a sense of happiness.

Self love, kindness, compassion, visualisation, affirmation and encouragement are supportive tools that can release and unlock your inner gifts of creativity and help you on the path to losing weight naturally.

**(c) The courage to be sensitive.**

Having the courage to be sensitive is one of the real gifts of our human experience. Many women who suffer from emotional eating and weight problems are sensitive or empathic in nature. They 'feel things' at a deep level and may also have strong intuitive, healing or spiritual abilities.

It is common to see these talents hidden behind excess weight for fear of judgment, ridicule and rejection. Excess weight then becomes a protective barrier to shelter them from the harshness of the world. This is usually because many women do not feel 'safe' expressing their sensitivity. Many of these fears are rooted in childhood.

Using emotional eating to soothe your feelings or burying them underneath excess weight does not get rid of them. Your emotions are energetically alive. If they are not expressed in some way, they do not go away, but simply move into a physical form and are stored in your body.

Your feelings really do matter. You do not need to hide your sensitivity behind emotional eating. You can bring much beauty to the world by having the courage to share your special talents.

**(d) The courage to go after your dreams.**

I commonly see women's dreams temporarily hidden or even lost underneath their excess weight.

To go after your dreams all you need to do is to make your courage bigger than your fear. When you draw on courage you can create the space in your life to uncover your deep desires. Like me, you may also discover that it is incredibly exciting to go after what you want.

This book is one that celebrates you following your dreams. It champions the idea that it is your purpose in life to identify and live the life of your dreams. For me, the lyric written by singer songwriter, Jack Johnson, "Don't let your dreams be dreams' captures this idea beautifully.

Imagine, spending your life living your dreams. What incredible things would you be doing? And how would those things make you feel? Know that it is possible for you to feel like this. It is your birthright to feel proud of yourself for what you have achieved in your life.

Do you remember what you wanted to do as a child? From a young age, all I wanted to do was to cook. My first job was in a cafe at the age of 12 years old. I scrubbed vegetables and washed dishes in exchange for the delight and joy of working in a cafe.

But as I got older, this dream faded as I replaced it with chasing University grades in my 4 year honours marketing degree. Luckily for me, I didn't allow this dream to disappear completely. Today I feel lucky that I can incorporate my love for creating delicious food into my personal life as well as my work. My husband and I have recently purchased a building that we are transforming into a yoga studio and vegetarian cafe in St Leonards by the sea in the United Kingdom. Here we plan to share our joint passion for yoga as well as healthy food.

Living life courageously, on your own terms, can enrich your life on many levels. Connect to what is actually important to you and that which gives your life meaning and purpose.

Use your feelings as your inner guidance system to help you connect more fully with living the life of your dreams. Your emotional eating is urging you to have the courage to make your dreams a reality. Having the courage to listen to your dreams and keep believing in them is an important part of your growth and healing journey.

**The courage to overcome emotional eating.**

When you have the courage to observe your emotional eating, it is a good sign that your old fear based emotions are ready to shift. Allow yourself to see how you can transform your emotional eating into your emotional healing.

In order to work with your feeling you must be willing to do something different. When you feel the craving to eat emotionally, rather than eating junk food, have the courage to look beneath the feeling. Keep listening to the deeper nutritional needs of your body. Cut back on stimulants and eat more green leafy vegetables to cleanse, energise and nourish yourself.

If you have an uncontrollable urge to emotionally eat it is okay. Just do it consciously. Observe what you are thinking and feeling before, during and after eating and make sure that you document it all in your journal. This is not an exercise in willpower, self-discipline or deprivation. It is an exercise in self-awareness.

Be kind and patient with yourself. This is very deep work. Honour yourself and give yourself lots of positive comments, encouragement and praise. You are an incredibly special human being and you deserve self love and support just as much as anyone else does.

## (2)  Address the root cause.

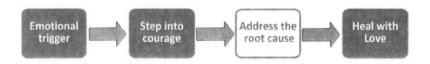

Your emotional eating is not the real problem; it is merely a symptom of it. Only when you address the root cause can you begin to heal the need to carry excess weight. When you address the root cause of your emotional eating, you are addressing the real problem.

The trouble with lap bands, weight loss pills or crash diets is that they don't address or heal the root cause of emotional eating. These so called 'solutions' only serve to mask the symptoms. To achieve long term weight loss results you are not looking for a 'band-aid solution' or any other kind of temporary relief or distraction from your pain.

### What is the root cause of emotional eating?

The 'root cause' of your emotional eating is an 'unhealed wound' that stems from your past. This wound may be the result of an isolated event or a series of interconnected events.

The pain of an unhealed wound can be opened or activated by some kind of trigger, stimulating the desire for emotional eating. These wounds may be something that you are already consciously working with or something that you haven't been ready to address until now.

The root cause of emotional eating is something that is unique to each individual. Just as each of our life experiences are unique, so too are the root causes for emotional eating.

The root cause can be something from a long time ago, and it can be something that is seemingly quite small. It does not need to be a big event. The root cause may be triggered by an unassuming comment from a family member or friend, or even a look or tone of voice that someone uses. Whenever you feel yourself being emotionally affected, simply notice how you feel and what is happening around you.

Finding the root cause is similar to putting together a jigsaw puzzle. Once you have enough pieces of the puzzle the root cause will reveal itself to you.

**Not feeling 'good enough'.**

Jacqui, a successful professional lady in her mid 50's, came to me for a breakthrough healing session.

Jacqui grew up not feeling good enough.  Her father made no secret about the fact that he had wanted a son.  Jacqui grew up trying to please her father.   She brought home straight A's from school and even became the youngest female to get into her Law school, but still she couldn't seem to impress him.

During the session, we worked on releasing the need for her father's approval and we replaced it with granting her self approval.   The visible shift in her outlook was incredible to behold.  No longer did she need to seek out peace and happiness through other people.  She was the one she had been looking for all along.

This simple awareness was a break-through moment for her and transformed how she felt about her life and her body.

**Addressing the root cause of my weight gain.**

When my doctors wanted me to take experimental medication without knowing what was wrong with me, I was stunned.  I didn't understand how they could possibly offer a solution without knowing what the real problem was.  This experience provided me with the motivation to look more deeply into my own life and discover the root cause of my emotional eating and health challenges for myself.

As I began to learn how to properly nourish my body with food, I became drawn to healing the emotional aspects of my life as well.  I read many books and attended courses that supported me on my quest for greater levels of self awareness.

When I began to look more deeply into my own life, I discovered that sitting at the root cause of my weight problems was an unhealed emotional wound.  This wound affected all aspects of my life.  Like Jacqui my emotional wound was a feeling of 'not being good enough'.

As I grew up, I can recall many occasions of 'not being good enough'.  My mind took these experiences as proof and evidence to support my perceived shortcomings.  As a result I often felt deeply embarrassed and ashamed of myself.

To compensate for this, I would try to win love and attention from those around me by being a 'good girl'.  I avoided 'rocking the boat' and kept my true feelings and self hidden. By my teenage years I had perfected the art of pleasing people.

Once I became aware of this old emotional wound I spent time observing and journaling my feelings, thoughts and food cravings. It was during this process I began to recognise my old and well-practiced childhood pattern revealing itself to me. Whenever something happened to make me feel like I was 'not good enough', I noticed that I would crave something sweet. Eating was my way of dealing with fear. Sugar soothed my emotions and feelings of inadequacy.

With time, I began to learn how to address the 'root cause' by looking for evidence in my life of when I did feel 'good enough'. I also discovered the importance of being true to myself. The more I was able to honour and express my own feelings, the less I craved sweet things.

Losing weight and overcoming my emotional eating was a process of learning how to accept myself. With practice and patience I was able to see that it was safe for me to be and express who I truly am. When I made these changes within myself, my world began to shift.

**Healing the root cause requires you to be honest with yourself.**

Addressing 'the root cause' of emotional eating requires you to be honest with yourself. The reason why honesty is so important is because addressing the root cause can often mean exploring 'the very thing' that you don't want to address. For some it may also be the thing that you don't want other people to know about as well.

It can be common for people to live in denial of their emotional pain. In fact, one of the main reasons that women may choose not to heal at the root cause, is if they think that it may be emotionally too painful to dig up their past. If this is the case for you, know that there are many different paths for healing emotional pain.

Understand that it is your old pain that holds you back from living your full potential. By consciously identifying what is going on emotionally for you, combined with a deeper understanding of the impact of emotional triggers, you can make a choice to break free of emotional eating for good. Healing emotional pain from your past is all part of your weight loss healing journey.

I did a breakthrough healing session with a woman who was struggling to lose weight. She told me all the things that she had tried to make changes to her life yet she thought she still was not making any progress. She said she was frustrated and confused. In the session, I asked her if it was okay for me to ask her subconscious mind something. She agreed. I asked, 'What is the one thing that you need to do to lose weight?' She immediately replied, 'I need to give up sugar.' Interestingly, the very next thing she said was, '...but I don't know if I can.' I assured her that she could, if she could find the right motivation.

We talked about what might motivate her. She said maybe if she approached it as if her life truly depended on giving up sugar that she might be able to do it. It was the break through she needed. In the coming weeks she substituted sugar for natural alternatives and couldn't believe how much better she felt.

By doing something that she didn't believe that she could do, she asked, 'If I can give up sugar, I wonder what else is possible for me in my life?' Simply by her asking this one question, I knew that she had hit an extremely powerful and transformative place in her life.

With a big dose of honesty, know that what is painful today, once healed, will free you to live the life you most desire.

**Healing the root cause requires you to be patient with yourself.**

Addressing the root cause of emotional eating can be challenging at times due to the complex and multi layered nature of the human experience.

Identifying and working with the root cause is not a quick fix. Given the integrative and holistic nature of this approach, it can require patience and kindness.

How long it will take, will vary from individual to individual. This is all part of the weight loss healing journey. The amount of time can vary due to how committed you are as well as how much inner work you have already done. This process will certainly take much longer than reaching for a bar of chocolate, tub of ice-cream or weight loss pill.

Know that change is possible for you when the pain of your emotional eating becomes greater than the perceived pain of addressing your emotional wound. When you choose to address it, you plant the seed for true and permanent transformation to occur.

Healing at the emotional root cause is the deepest healing work that you can do. Take things at your own pace. Know that you can progress at a speed that feels comfortable for you, particularly if you feel emotionally raw at any stage during this process. Be patient and give yourself the time, space and support that you need.

**Everything is being perfectly revealed to you.**

It can be common for women to heal the root cause of their emotional eating only to wish that they had done it sooner. Just trust that everything is being revealed to you at the perfect time.

Your higher self is aware of the root cause of your emotional eating. As you move along your journey, ask your higher self to reveal any hidden patterns to you so that you can heal and release them.

It is the natural desire of your feminine spirit to feel powerful, to believe, to nourish, to trust and to powerfully love yourself, others and life completely. Being connected to your inner wisdom, power and strength will allow you and your self-confidence, your self-esteem and your sense of worth to flourish.

I know that overcoming emotional eating can be challenging at times. I also know how rewarding it can be when you have the courage to look within. Creating true health happens when you address the root cause to rebalance any disharmony within the body, mind and spirit. Doing so creates vibrant health along with self confidence and happiness.

I deeply honour you for having the willingness and courage to work at this level. As you move forward, celebrate every little break through and keep extending love and kindness to yourself.

**(3) Heal with Love.**

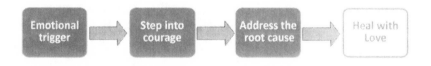

At the core of your being exists an incredible ability to heal your emotional eating with Love.

Healing with Love is a process of gently releasing the obstacles and obstructions that prevent you from deeply loving and accepting who you are at your core. When you heal with Love, you release the stuck energy that has prevented you from living in your natural flow.

This gentle healing process involves embracing the Love and light that you already have within you. You do not need to do anything at all to be worthy and deserving of Love.

You are beautiful just as you are. You are a magnificent being on a miraculous journey of discovery and no one deserves Love more than you do. An affirmation that can help you embody this awareness is *'I am worthy and deserving of Love.'*

This type of healing focuses upon bringing harmony and balance back to the whole person by honouring the body, mind, emotions and spirit.

Healing with Love allows you to reconnect with your true self. You are whole and complete exactly as you are. You do not need to search for things outside of yourself.

Acknowledging your wholeness will reduce your desire to emotionally eat and as a result will bring you an increased sense of confidence and self assurance.

On my own weight loss journey, learning how to love and accept myself was a huge challenge that I had to face and overcome. Having healed my own emotional eating and weight problems, I know that it is possible for anyone with the courage to look within and start healing with Love.

In my workshops, retreats and yoga classes as well as my private healing sessions, I help women to gently remove the barriers that hold them back from being able to love and accept themselves fully.

When you navigate your way back to your own centre you are healing your life with the power of Love. Be kind and compassionate towards the parts of you that are ready to heal.

Even if you feel that you are not ready to love and accept yourself as you are just yet, start to gently open to the possibility that one day soon you will be able to.

When you begin to Love yourself in this way you set the scene for the most remarkable things to unfold in your life. The power of this positive energy is so embracing that it will overflow into all areas of your life and indeed, everything that you do.

This is a very special time for you. See your emotional eating as a call to release your fears, let go of your past and step into your true power.

**Healing tools to end emotional eating.**

There are many different types of healing tools, techniques and modalities available today to help you transform and heal your emotional eating patterns.

The healing tools recommended in this section can help you to gently heal old pain, release your past and move beyond your current fears. Just notice within yourself, which ones you feel intuitively drawn towards.

Healing tools will help you to gain clarity, consciousness and awareness of your emotions and your resulting actions. They help to integrate and align both your body and mind, so that you can break free of your emotional eating and move forward in your life.

Energy moves when you create an outlet for your emotions and self expression. When you let go and express your feelings using these healing tools, you will be able to move any stuck energy. Using these tools will help you to interrupt, release and heal your old habits and emotional patterns.

There are many options for healing. Choose emotional healing tools that inspire and energise you. Overcoming emotional eating may require using one or even a combination of these healing tools.

Here is a list of some gentle healing tools that will help you to release fear and let go of the past. The list is not an exhaustive one but think of it as a good place to get started on your emotional healing journey.

To find out more about each one, look them up on the internet and notice which healing modalities resonate with you. Think of these healing tools as spiritual and emotional nutrition for your soul.

**Physical release**

- Eating real foods
- Breathing
- Walking
- Healing yoga
- 5 Rhythms dancing
- Rebounding
- Massage
- Colonic irrigation

## Mental release

- Life coaching
- Counselling
- Neuro-linguistic programming (NLP)
- Voice dialogue
- Parts integration
- Writing or journalling
- Emotional Freedom Technique (EFT)
- Kinesiology (muscle testing)
- Touch For Health (TFH)
- Bowen therapy
- Family constellation
- Inner child healing
- Acupuncture
- Hypnosis
- Chi-gong
- Tai-chi
- Reiki
- Shiatsu

## Spiritual connection

- Affirmations
- Visualisations
- Meditation
- Vibrational healing
- Energetic healing

## Creative connection

- Art classes
- Pottery classes
- Singing classes
- Drumming classes
- Improvisation and acting classes

## You can heal emotional eating.

*"Healing takes courage, and we all have courage, even if we have to dig a little to find it."*

*~ Tori Amos*

To heal your emotional eating is to make friends with your emotions. When you befriend your emotions, you can allow them to guide your body and life back into balance.

Every emotion is an invaluable part of the human experience, yet as a society we tend to label our emotions as either 'good' or 'bad'. The reality is that all your emotions are invaluable and provide a rich texture of life experience. Consider that each emotion holds an exquisite message for you on how to orientate your life moving forward.

Your emotions are your personal guidance system. Think of emotions as your very own sign posts to steer you along your weight loss healing journey.

Feeling an emotion and expressing it through tears, laughter or even yawning is a sign that stuck energy is gently being released from your body. When this happens, your life force energy can start to mobilise and flow freely again.

Your emotions are always calling you back to the inner voice of your heart. It is here where you will be able to access the awareness, knowledge and self healing that you are seeking. Your heart is always whispering gently to you to honour yourself and be the best you can be.

When you are living in alignment with the truth of your heart, you are plugging back into your own energy source and restoring a natural balance to your life. When you turn your gaze outwards, it is very easy for your energy system to become over extended and out of balance.

When you are open to learning and growing, you begin to understand how your emotions are there to guide you to focus your energy in the right direction. Turning your gaze inwards in this way will enable you to further evolve on your weight loss healing journey.

When you change how you treat yourself, this naturally affects the way that you treat other people. When you treat yourself and others with kindness, love and compassion, you will find yourself being treated in the same way too!

I remember working with one client, who couldn't understand why people treated her with anger. In her own words she said it was like, 'the whole world was against her'. Initially, she thought that there was something wrong with the people that she met but over time she kept noticing the same pattern appearing. She began to wonder why this was happening to her and if there might be something that she was projecting into the world. As we worked together, she was able to release a lot of anger that she had been unconsciously holding inside her body since she was a little girl. Much of this anger was directed at her mother who she described as 'mean, evil and controlling.'

I caught up with her a few weeks after our session and she said that she couldn't believe how nice people had been treating her. She told me that now she understood that she had been sending angry negative vibes towards herself and this had spilled out into the world. Upon releasing her past, she realised that the old, angry energy that she had been previously emitting had been positively transformed.

**Learning how to say 'no'.**

An essential part of healing your emotional eating is learning how to say 'no'. Saying 'no' is a great way to interrupt deeply entrenched behavioural patterns.

Saying 'no' means learning how to set boundaries for yourself. Many people, particularly women, struggle with saying 'no' because they like to keep others happy.

Living to please others is a certain road to a life of misery. It can also seriously impact your weight loss progress. You can find plenty of ways to say 'no' in a manner that is kind and polite.

Your happiness comes from living in integrity with your own values. Know that when you say 'no', others will appreciate your clarity and the fact that you speak your truth. It will also give people the assurance that when you say 'yes', that you really mean it.

Below are some examples of saying 'no':

Social pressure around food:

- *'No I don't want to eat that, thank you.'*
- *'No thanks, I'm fine. I've already eaten but thanks for asking'*
- *'No, I'd prefer it if we didn't order a pizza and chips.'*

Setting clear boundaries with family, friends and work colleagues:

- *'No I can't work late today. I'm attending my dance class.'*
- *'No I'm not able to do that for you. Maybe ask Jen if she can?'*
- *'No I really don't want to watch television tonight'*

**Learn to say 'yes' to yourself.**

Saying yes to yourself is something that can be totally life transforming, particularly if you spend a lot of time attending to the needs of others, whilst putting your own needs aside.

Saying 'yes' to yourself is about learning how to honour your own needs. If you are not accustomed to doing things just for you, start small.

Consider the many different ways you could say 'yes' to yourself. Possible options could include going to a movie, having a massage or even booking a yoga retreat. Anything that helps you to relax and move emotion in your body assists you to release stress naturally from your life.

What would happen if you started putting yourself first? What if you gave yourself permission to say 'yes' and follow your hearts desires?

Do you remember Elizabeth Gilbert from the book, 'Eat Pray Love'? It was only by saying yes to herself that she could connect with the inner courage to follow her own path, which saw her end her relationship with her boyfriend and then travel to 3 countries, including Italy, India and Bali. This led to her 'finding' herself, falling in love and subsequently writing a best-selling novel.

A friend of mine shares a wonderful story of how she used to live her life trying to please everyone else around her. She tried her hardest to be everything that she thought a great wife should be. She was a Super mum to her 3 boys and a career girl earning £200,000+ a year, but she was also 30 pounds overweight because of an emotional eating pattern that she had slipped into.

To an 'outsider' she said that her life looked picture perfect. She had pursued everything that she had been told would bring happiness; she had a great family, an expensive house with a 2 acre farm as well as huge career success. She said that despite everything, on the inside she felt like she was dying. It was only by saying 'no' to everyone else and 'yes' to herself that she was able to be true to her own desires and pave her own path to happiness.

Today, she is a writer who inspires people to say yes to themselves and follow the truth of their hearts. Once she started living life on her own terms, her emotional eating disappeared, her waist line decreased and her sense of dress changed as well.

Routinely people comment on her levels of energy and youthfulness, thinking that she is 10 years younger than she really is.

Once you feel comfortable saying 'yes' to yourself, begin to notice when you say 'yes' to others, especially when you would rather say 'no'. With time you will build the courage and inner confidence to express your true feelings with not only yourself, but with others as well.

Saying 'yes' to yourself and really communicating your own needs will leave you feeling more self-confident, self-assured and empowered.

**Self-awareness is key.**

When you embark upon your journey to heal your emotional eating, self awareness is key. Becoming aware of how, when and why you are eating emotionally, allows you to start making different choices for yourself. Know that there are other ways that you can deal with your feelings that will leave you feeling healthy, strong and empowered.

If you have not been taught how to express your true feelings, at first doing so may feel strange.

I remember how tricky it was for me when I first began to express myself. I was worried that people might not like me. It felt scary and unnatural.

If you can relate to this all you need to do is keep practicing. Learning how to express your feelings is a skill which becomes easier with repetition. You will get better and stronger the more you practice.

Believe and know that this is something that you can do.

If you are an emotional eater, developing awareness of your real feelings is a powerful step to healing. Self awareness is the golden key that unlocks the door to losing weight naturally.

# Chapter Seven – Starting Your Healing Journey

*"Happiness cannot come from without. It must come from within."*

*~ Helen Keller*

## Be willing to change.

*"Change is the essence of life. Be willing to surrender what you are for what you could become."*

*~ Author unknown*

When you set off on your healing journey it is important that you become willing to change.

A willingness to change is something that comes from within you. You don't need permission or any special talent, skills or abilities, just an internal desire to improve the quality of your life.

Being willing to change means having an openness to seeing and doing things differently. It means allowing yourself to experiment so that you are able to uncover new and improved approaches for living. It means being willing to 'let go of the old' so that you can 'open to the new'.

### The mantra of change.

It is important to realise that you do not need to transform your entire life overnight - far from it. Often it is the subtle changes in either your outlook or approach that can make all the difference.

When I set off on my weight loss journey, I didn't even know if change was possible. I grew up in a small country town in New Zealand where pretty much everything seemed to stay the same. I didn't have any role models that could help me to see that my life could be anything other than what it was.

After my health break down, I knew that I wanted my life to be different but I didn't know where to start. I didn't know anyone who had managed to successfully lose weight let alone change the course of their life.

One day when I was pondering this dilemma, a simple phrase entered my consciousness.

*'I am willing to change'.*

I was so taken by the little phrase that I immediately whispered it again to myself. These five words seemed to hold such an immense power, so I repeated them again a little louder this time. It was hard to really know exactly what was going on at the time, but I did feel as if something had profoundly shifted within me. And so I repeated the phrase again and again.

I used this phrase many times over the course of my weight loss healing journey. In fact I still use it today any time I want to change something in my life. These five words are immensely powerful. You can repeat them as many times as you like. Try saying the words aloud to yourself right now.

*'I am willing to change'.*

Feel the strength, energy and power of these words. Repeat this mantra anytime you experience resistance to change. You will find these words particularly powerful any time you are feeling blocked, frustrated or confused.

If you are in a public place reading this book and feel a little self conscious you can always try writing these words down on a piece of paper instead.

This one statement can conquer fear, anxiety, uncertainty and doubt. You can connect to your inner power whenever you feel like you want to, just by repeating these words.

Being willing to change can open up a whole new range of possibilities in your life and can be a real catalyst on your path to healing.

**Use this book to help you change.**

As you have been making your way through this book, I have been inviting you to review and upgrade the different aspects of your life, in particular your physical, mental and emotional practices.

Change can be a scary thing for many people but it doesn't have to be. You can choose to feel safe as you step forward to transform your old ways. This approach is a powerful way to release fear and access the magic that is waiting to be revealed in your life.

There is a natural universal intelligence guiding and supporting your highest evolution. Connect with this awareness. Welcome new people, resources and opportunities into your life and allow them to support your healing so that you can lose weight naturally.

The way that I personally look at change these days, is just as a gentle way to release my old ways, so I can bring something more exciting into my life. This approach was incredibly useful to me on my weight loss healing journey. I have also used it, with great success, transforming other areas of my life as well and I know that you can too.

---

# Exercise: Be willing to change.

Being willing to change is an important step to creating and connecting to your inner world. Try the following exercise and write down your experiences in your journal.

Stay sitting where you are and then gently close your eyes

1. Now, quietly say to yourself, '*I am willing to change*'

   ...............................................................

2. Notice how you feel when you say this

   ...............................................................

3. Write down your feelings

   ...............................................................

---

## Accept where you are.

*"There are two primary choices in life: to accept conditions as they exist, or accept the responsibility for changing them."*

*~Denis Waitley*

If you want to lose weight naturally it is imperative that you accept where you are. It doesn't matter if you have a little weight to lose or a lot, where you are right now is the perfect place for you to begin your weight loss journey.

When I was really struggling with my weight, I remember thinking how easy my life would be if I was just 'somewhere else' or 'someone else'. Years of this kind of thinking only ever resulted in constant tears and me feeling sorry for myself.

It was only when I was able to accept the fact that I was '60 pounds overweight', that I was able to begin the journey back to regaining my health and my perfect weight. As challenging as it was for me to see at the time, it was essential to realise that this was the perfect place that I needed to re-create my life from.

**Acceptance is the doorway to transformation.**

The only place you can ever be is exactly where you are. Accepting where you are is part of your challenge on the weight loss and healing journey. When you accept where you are, you have a very real chance of gaining the valuable life lessons necessary to move forward in the direction of your dreams.

Can you imagine looking at a map and knowing exactly where you want to end up, but having no idea of where you currently are? It would be a pretty futile exercise. This is the very reason why most public maps have the big red arrow that says 'you are here'. It is only when you 'know where you are' and 'know where you want to go' that you are able to start charting a course to your desired destination.

**Whatever you resist... persists.**

Have you heard the saying, 'Whatever you resist persists'? I can guarantee that if you resist being overweight, then there is a very good chance that you will continue to be overweight. The very opposite of resistance and the key to losing weight for good, is acceptance.

How would your life be different if you just accepted where you are without any excuses, stories or self judgement? What would happen if you stopped fighting with your body and embraced it instead?

Accepting where you are is not about rolling over and trying to live with being overweight forever. Accepting where you are is about bringing the focus of your life into the present moment, so that you can move forward powerfully.

All of your combined life experiences have brought you to where you are right now including your setbacks, your struggles, as well as all of your successes. Just as the butterfly first had to be a caterpillar, you are here in the present moment ready to transform into the highest possibility of yourself.

This moment is the gateway to the next moment and it is calling you to step up and be who you really are. You are being called to express your true self. This is your journey of transformation and the right time for you to get started is now.

When I look back on my own weight loss journey, it is easy for me to see why I struggled with my weight for so long. The simple reason being, I couldn't be the person I am today without confronting and healing my own weight loss demons. It was through this challenge that I have been able to create the life of freedom that I enjoy today. It has also provided me with the knowledge and direct experience to help other women to go on their own healing journey to lose weight naturally.

**Removing old layers.**

Losing weight for good is a healing journey of self discovery, that strips back all the old layers that cover over and hide who you really are.

Just as it takes time to become overweight, removing the old layers takes time too. Know that this time is a real gift. It will give you the opportunity to gather new understandings and integrate them into your life. Use this time to deepen your awareness of the physical, mental and emotional aspects of yourself.

If you are ready to change, then there is a good chance that some of your life strategies are no longer working for you. There is no point hiding behind these old patterns or excuses any more. Let them dissolve to reveal the magnificence of who you really are.

**Being overweight will become a distant memory.**

Learning to heal yourself and lose weight naturally is a journey that will transform you from within. You are moving forward to a new you. There is something amazing on the other side of your weight challenge. Even if you don't know exactly what it is, know that it will be something quite magical.

Accept your body as it is and love it unconditionally for being the vehicle through which you can experience this thing we call life. The struggle against it is futile. Each and every day find new things to acknowledge and appreciate.

If you can learn to accept where you are on your healing journey and allow yourself to move forward from this place, being overweight will soon become a distant memory.

# Commit to your healing journey.

*"Love is always the answer to healing of any sort."*

*~ Louise Hay*

After many years of studying human behaviour, I can tell you that there is a huge difference between someone who is 'committed' to doing something versus someone who is 'not quite sure'.

When you are 'not quite sure' about your commitment to self-healing and losing weight, you are far more likely to be open to the influence of your environment and the thoughts of other people. There are two very basic forms of weight loss commitments that I will explore in this section: 'short term commitments' and 'long term commitments'.

**Short term weight loss commitments.**

The dieting industry is obsessed with luring women into making short term commitments with their health and their weight.

These short term approaches are one of the main reasons why 95% of all diets fail. Most diets are specifically designed to keep you on the weight loss tread mill for life and why most women end up putting on more weight than they lose when dieting.

One of the main reasons why most diets fail is because they take a 'crash' approach to health and weight loss. Here are some typical magazine headlines encouraging women to make short term dieting commitments:

- 'Shed 7 pounds in 7 days'
- 'Lose your bingo wings fast'
- 'Drop a dress size before the weekend'
- 'Look fab this festive season'
- 'Get your college body back'
- 'Summer + Bikini = You'

**Long term weight loss commitments.**

The key to losing weight naturally is in making sustainable long term commitments to yourself and to your body.

Making a commitment to healing your body and losing weight naturally requires a shift in your mindset and lifestyle. It is easy to do when you take a long-term, holistic and healing approach that honours your body-mind connection as well as the hopes and aspirations of your heart and your spirit.

How do you personally feel when you contemplate the following possibilities?

(a) Losing a few extra pounds this month; versus

(b) Healing your weight loss problems for good

When I was overweight I didn't even know that losing weight permanently was an option. It felt like I had struggled with my weight all my life. From seeing weight struggles of celebrities in newspapers and magazines, I had always just assumed that even if I did lose weight, that it would continue to be an ongoing life long battle for me to keep it off.

One thing that can help you make the necessary commitment to losing weight is to imagine how incredible you would feel if you never had another weight problem again.

### The benefits of making the commitment of losing weight for good.

Here are some of the benefits that I have personally experienced:

- I feel confident and self assured about myself and my body.
- I no longer worry what other people think when I eat in public.
- I can always find clothes in my size when I go shopping.
- I can wear bikinis at the beach, without feeling self conscious.
- I no longer seek validation and approval from anyone else.
- I feel deeply loved and accepted in my personal relationships.

The real gift of losing weight naturally is feeling differently about yourself. Losing weight for good is about creating a loving and harmonious relationship with yourself.

Lydia committed herself fully to healing and changing her life. Along her journey she has experimented with different ways of eating, from vegetarian, vegan and raw diets, arriving at a place of balance and love for her body. Today she follows a simple eating philosophy by listening to her body, eating food that she feels intuitively drawn towards. On average she thinks that this is about 80% real, whole foods and 20% other foods.

When I asked Lydia what she thinks is her secret to successfully healing her body, she said that the most important thing has been to make a profound commitment to her own health and wellbeing. Along the way she has learned how to deeply value herself and respect her body.

**Only you can make the commitment to losing weight.**

No one else can do it for you.  Losing weight is a commitment that you have to make to yourself for yourself.

If you are ready to lose weight for good, then make that commitment to yourself now.  Life is far too short to spend another day agonizing over your weight.

When you commit to losing weight permanently you will transform your life for the better. Your connection to your inner wisdom and power will strengthen and you will be well on your way to creating the best possible you.

---

# Exercise:  Commit to losing weight for good.

How committed are you to losing weight for good?  In your journal answer the following questions.

1.  Are you ready to make changes in your life?

     ...................................................................

2.  Are you ready to experiment with different foods?

     ...................................................................

3.  Are you ready to move your body in ways that feel good?

     ...................................................................

4.  Are you ready to lose weight for good?

     ...................................................................

# Find your 'BIG why'.

*"It's kind of fun to do the impossible."*

*~ Walt Disney*

Having a 'BIG why' is the lightening rod that will ignite your long term weight loss success.

Your 'BIG why' is your compelling motivation for losing weight for good. It should fill you with excitement, energy and new possibilities for your life. When you find your 'BIG why', the whole process of losing weight will become so much easier for you.

Before you can uncover your 'BIG why', it is often useful to compile a detailed list of all the different possible reasons why you want to lose weight. Try to make the list as exhaustive as possible. Add every reason that comes into your mind no matter how small or insignificant it may seem.

When you connect with your reasons for change, you massively increase your ability to achieve long term weight loss. You will also start to build the neurological pathways necessary for your brain to create successful behavioural change.

Having lots of reasons why you want to lose weight has the dual purpose of helping you to interrupt old beliefs, habits and patterns as well as build clarity and motivation. The more reasons you can give your brain why losing weight is important to you, the more compelling your weight loss journey will become.

### Finding reasons to lose weight.

One of the things that I discovered on my own weight loss journey, was that my desire for losing weight in and of itself was never going to be a big enough reason for permanent weight loss.

Just as excess weight is never the 'real problem', losing weight is never the 'real solution'. I knew that I needed to dig a little deeper to discover my true motivations for losing weight.

When you discover your true motivations for losing weight, old mindsets of 'having to go on a diet' will feel tired and outdated. Instead your motivation and desire to change will be supercharged from within.

To find out my real reasons for losing weight, I asked myself the following simple question...

*'What will losing weight really give me?'*

I took out a piece of paper and pen and wrote down everything that entered my mind. I wrote and wrote until my hand couldn't write anymore.

Some of my reasons for wanting to lose weight included:

1.  To heal my body and regain my health and well being.
2.  To have more energy and vitality.
3.  To release the excess toxicity from my body.
4.  To feel comfortable eating in public.
5.  To feel less self conscious when I go clothes shopping.
6.  To rebuild my self confidence.
7.  To have a body I can be proud of.
8.  To develop an intimate relationship with someone special.
9.  To grow my circle of friends.
10. To attract more opportunities into my life.
11. To live an active life and travel the world.
12. To feel more comfortable on aeroplanes.
13. To be able to wear fitted jeans.
14. To wear swimsuits and not feel embarrassed.
15. To buy lingerie and feel sexy wearing it.
16. To increase my chances of finding inspiring work.
17. To begin breathing properly by healing my asthma.
18. To clear my skin of eczema.
19. To make my friends and family proud.
20. To see what I could achieve when I set my mind to it.

**Clarifying your 'BIG why.'**

Once you have finished compiling a list of all the many reasons why you want to lose weight (make sure you write down at least 20), take a moment to read back over your list. Highlight any items that really strike an emotional chord for you (ideally your refined list should have at least 3-5 items on it).

From this refined list, allow yourself to go deeper by expanding what each reason actually means to you. Write at least a paragraph (or more if you like) for each item.

For example, if one of your highlighted reasons is to feel comfortable eating in public, then describe in as much detail as possible what this will mean for you in your life.

From going deeper in this way, not only will you become more fully attuned to your motivations, you will also be able to uncover your 'BIG why' (be open to being very surprised by what you discover).

Once you have uncovered your 'BIG why', really allow yourself to experience the true emotional potency behind it. By doing this you will allow it to become anchored into your being.

With your 'BIG why' you have the secret ingredient to keep you focused and on track with your weight loss goals. It will provide you with the sustained motivation you need, as well as the inner strength necessary to transform your life for the better. Your 'BIG why' will give you the courage and strength to keep going, even when times feel difficult or challenging.

With your 'BIG why' to spur you on, you are guaranteed of weight loss success. Allow it to be your motivational 'hot button' that you can call upon any time you need.

**Uncovering my own 'BIG why' for losing weight.**

On my own journey, my 'BIG why' surprisingly found me when I least expected it.

When I was really struggling with my weight, there was a part of me that questioned whether it was ever going to be possible. After all of my failed dieting attempts, I certainly had more than enough proof to suggest that losing weight, at best, was going to be a very difficult endeavour.

Despite the overwhelming evidence I had accumulated on my inability to lose weight, for some strange reason a small voice kept appearing inside my head with the question:

*'But what if you could lose weight?'*

At first, I did my best to just ignore the voice so I could get on with the task of accepting the seemingly obvious fact that I was going to be overweight forever.  But it persisted.  I sat with this little voice momentarily and then swiftly concluded that my life would be much easier without it and dismissed it.

Over the coming weeks and months I did my best to extinguish the voice, but no matter how hard I tried, it kept chiming in when I least expected it with it's silly little question.

*'But what if you could lose weight?'*

After a period of resisting the voice I finally relented.  I decided that if this little voice could still believe in me, despite my obvious weaknesses and failings, then maybe, just maybe losing weight was possible.

Not only that, if it was prepared to make a stand for me, even in my darkest moments, then maybe it was the inspiration I had been searching for all along.

As strange and unexpected as it seemed, I decided to make friends with this small voice.  Very soon this little voice became my weight loss champion and my 'BIG why'.

Any time I felt disheartened or ready to give up, I instinctively thought about the faith and courage of that small voice deep inside of me and I instantly found the courage and strength to keep going.

**Use your 'BIG why' to create a bold new vision for your life.**

Once I started to lose weight, I wanted to keep going.  I wondered with anticipation and excitement what kind of life was waiting for me on the other side of my weight loss.  I was driven by a burning desire to keep learning more about healthy food, as well as fun and interesting ways to move and connect with my body.

My 'BIG why' filled me with inspiration and it gave me the confidence to create a bold new vision for my life.  It revealed that not only was it possible for me to lose weight, but also that my life could be radically different to the way it had been.

It encouraged me to contemplate what my life could be like if I lost my excess weight. New thoughts and ideas entered my mind. I wondered about things such as *'Who could I be if I lost weight?'*, 'what new things would I be able to pursue in my life that I don't right now?' and 'what new and exciting possibilities would open for me and my life?'

I remember being really moved by this quote from Lao Tzu at that time: *'When I let go of what I am, I become what I might be.'*

Whatever your own personal 'BIG why' is, allow it to create a bold new vision of what is possible for you and your life. Allow it to shape the person that you are in the process of becoming and act as a motivational force for tremendous change in your life.

Discovering your 'BIG why' will help you to live in alignment with your dreams. It will enable you to tap into your inner strength and the potent motivational power that is currently living dormant within you.

When you have a big enough reason, your body will let you know. Things will just be different in your life. Different people will begin to show up. You will make different choices for yourself. You will say different things. You will think, dream, visualise and literally create a new life for yourself.

You already have everything you need to start upon your journey to heal and lose weight naturally. With your 'BIG why' to motivate you, you will be able to do anything that you put your mind to.

# Exercise:  Find your 'BIG why'.

In your journal, answer the following questions to clearly identify what your 'BIG why' is and how you can use it to motivate you to start your own weight loss healing journey.

1.  What new feelings do you want to create in your life?

    ...............................................................................

2.  What old energy are you ready to release from your life?

    ...............................................................................

3.  What new opportunities do you want to create in your life?

    ...............................................................................

## Take responsibility.

*"The willingness to accept responsibility for one's own life is the source from which self-respect springs."*

*~ Joan Didion*

One of the most effective things your can do on your healing journey is to take responsibility for your weight and your physical health. If you don't take responsibility for your health, someone else will.  The unfortunate thing is that they may not have your best interests at heart.

Many women struggle with their weight for the very simple fact that they have given responsibility for their health over to someone else.

Taking responsibility means making your own decisions about the direction of your health and your life.  This means becoming very clear about what you will and won't do. It also means doing your own research and becoming aware of the steps necessary for you to create vibrant health.

## The business of weight loss.

Companies that operate on a profit-driven approach, without care or concern for the greater social implications of their actions, will always pursue their own interests, often at the expense of your health.  As sad as it seems, there are organisations that have a vested financial interest in keeping you distracted, uninformed and overweight.

In our prevailing western culture of 'bigger is better', there are many organisations that value profits over working towards creating a healthy and sustainably functioning society.  What's worse is that they will often invest vast amounts of money into advertising and marketing to try and convince you otherwise.

Unfortunately the real truth remains hidden from the public.  It is this 'profit at all costs' model that is a large contributing factor in the ever increasing numbers of people that are sick, tired, fat and also broke.

Today many fast food restaurants compete solely on price.  To sell food competitively they have to buy and source the cheapest ingredients possible.  Stop and think about it. If you are buying a burger for one or two pounds, what kind of 'real food' can possibly be in it?  Eating at fast food restaurants supports theses business practices whilst damaging your health.

In most profit driven organisations, making the cheapest products, increasing shareholder value and maximising the bottom line is the primary motive for making business decisions.  If they can make a cheaper product they will, even if it has a negative impact on your health and the greater environment.

Taking back responsibility for your own health is about saying 'no' to this type of behaviour by consciously withdrawing your financial support.  You can no longer afford to hand your body, health and wealth over to organisations that think that profits are more important than your personal well being.

The good news is that we are living in a world that is in a very powerful process of evolution.   There are increasing numbers of inspired and ethical food companies that are stepping up to guide the planet back to one of health and sustainability.

**Take responsibility for your purchasing decisions.**

When you take responsibility for your health and start supporting ethical companies, that have a genuine interest in co-creating a better world, you start to become part of the solution.

As more and more people raise their level of awareness and take responsibility for their own health, companies are coming under increasing levels of pressure to become responsible for their actions.

Whether you like it or not, each time you open your wallet you are voting for the kind of world that you live in. Each pound that you spend is a vote in favour of your health and wellbeing or a vote against it. By taking responsibility for your purchasing decisions, you will not only improve your own health, but you are helping to foster and finance a happier and healthier world.

The most important thing to realise is that you do have a choice. When I woke up to this fact, I started making different choices for myself. I also got inspired to encourage other people to do the same.

You simply must discover the truth for yourself. Begin by learning from people who have achieved the health results you are after. Don't believe what they say. Take it and then test it for yourself. If something resonates with you, investigate it further. If it doesn't, move on and find something that does.

**Take responsibility for your health.**

Taking responsibility for your health begins with getting proactive, asking questions and demanding truthful answers.

Some great ways that you can kick off this process is by reading food labels, asking how and where your food is produced, questioning food marketing and advertising, shopping in alignment with what you truly value and educating yourself about 'real food' and nutrition.

As you start to take responsibility for yourself and your actions, work alongside someone that you trust. Find a natural health practitioner that will encourage you to connect back to your own body and support you in making more empowered decisions about your food and lifestyle choices.

Getting educated about your health can be simple. You don't have to be a medical doctor or a dietician. There are loads of small, easy things that you can do that will result in natural weight loss.

Always remember that what is true for someone else may not be true for you. The one thing you can trust is that your body always knows your truth. You simply cannot delegate your health to others and expect to stay healthy. The only person in the world that has the right to except full responsibility for your health and wellness is you.

# Step out of your 'comfort zone'.

*"Life loses its meaning when we get stuck in our comfort zone".*

*~ M. K. Soni*

If you want to heal your life and lose weight for good, sooner or later you are going to have to step outside of what is already comfortable for you.

Living within your comfort zone means to live within a limited set of routines, parameters or behaviours.

Living with this kind of orientation can produce a fairly predictable level of performance and life experience, albeit in many cases, with results that are far from desirable.

Be aware that living safely is very restrictive. It is often said, 'the safe path is not always the safe path.'

It is worth noting that it is your consistent comfort zone behavioural patterns that keep you from losing weight permanently and naturally.

Some classic 'comfort zone' behaviours include:

- Wanting to lose weight but being afraid to try something different.
- Eating the same coffee and muffin on the way to work.
- Eating lunch at your desk more often than not.
- Eating dinner in front of the television when you get home at night.
- Drinking more than you should because that's what you have always done.

It is important to realise that if you stay living from within your comfort zone, there is a very good chance that you will keep getting the same kind of results in your life.


**Fear of the unknown.**


The biggest factor that keeps people living inside the prison of their comfort zone is the 'fear of the unknown'.

For most women, this fear of the unknown is largely an 'unexamined fear'. These fears become even more acute if you are someone who worries about getting things wrong or what other people will think about you.

Now let me get one thing straight. There is absolutely nothing wrong with experiencing fear. Fear is a natural part of being human. It is only when these fears hold you back from living the life that you desire, that it is worth taking the time to examine them.

The key is to let your fears catalyse you into facing your weight loss challenges head on. By trusting yourself and cultivating the courage to take risks, you can start to shift those unwanted pounds.

On my own weight loss journey there were many occasions where I had to face my personal fears and step outside of what was comfortable for me. It has been amazing to witness how many of my fears have disappeared simply from having the willingness and courage to confront them.

Being okay to sit in the space of uncertainty, is the key to changing your relationship with fear. I love the Woody Allen quote, '*If you want to make God laugh, show him your plan.*' This saying reminds me of how life is always wanting to move us towards something more meaningful and fulfilling if we can only move out of our comfort zones.

This is what happened to Jennifer, a client who was ready to confront her deepest fears and navigate the path back to her true self.


**Waiting for approval before taking action.**


Jennifer was already a young, passionate and very successful medical doctor working in the slums of South Africa. Despite the success she had achieved in her professional life, her weight as well as her general state of health was becoming an increasing concern for her.

She wanted to shed her excess pounds but in a natural and holistic way, without drugs or surgery. Having studied, trained and worked within the medical field she was very present to the influence and orientation of her education. While she was immersed in the field of modern medicine, she could readily see that it did not offer her the solution she was looking for.

For professional as well as personal reasons her heart was calling her to study nutrition and natural medicine, but she felt afraid to take the necessary steps forward for fear of ridicule. As we talked more about her feelings she identified that she was concerned about what other people would say, particularly her family and her work colleagues.

Once she connected with her inner power she was able to move into the drivers' seat of her life. She committed taking her life in the direction that felt true for her and let go of the fears that were holding her back from living a life aligned with her values.

She recognised that the medical world had become her comfort zone and she was being called to explore what lay beyond it in the field of complementary medicine.

While she still felt some fear about taking the steps forward to expand her mind and studies on health, healing and nutrition, she recognised that she must stop waiting for the approval of other people and instead give herself the permission she was seeking.


**Breaking free of your comfort zone.**


To break free of your comfort zone it is essential that you start to experiment with doing new things so that you can begin to create new habits and behaviours.

With each small step you take outside of your comfort zone it may initially feel a little uncomfortable. After a while this will eventually become what is comfortable for you and in the process you will have totally expanded who you are as a human being.

To break out of your comfort zone start experimenting. Small ways to begin include:

- Try new foods and 'healthy options'.
- Brush your teeth with your opposite hand.

- Travel a different way to work each day.
- Take the stairs instead of the lift.
- Do something new each day that scares or excites you.

When you have had plenty of practice with the small stuff, you can start experimenting with things like jobs or relationships that are no longer working for you.

When you step outside of your comfort zone, you will find yourself better able to start taking the risks necessary to grow and expand as a human being.

With each risk that you take you will feel yourself growing in confidence and it will propel forward along your weight loss healing journey.

---

# Exercise:  Break out of your comfort zone.

1. Think of something that you have always wanted to do

...............................................................................

2.  What is one baby step that you can take towards it?

...............................................................................

3.  Do it and in your journal write down what you experience

...............................................................................

---

## Learn to trust yourself.

*"As soon as you trust yourself, you will know how to live."*

*~ Johann Wolfgang von Goethe*

A big part of the weight loss healing journey is learning how to trust yourself and your body. Much of my weight loss success came from being willing to cultivate trust in myself and in my body's natural healing ability.

Over the past few years I have helped many women, both in private healing sessions and in workshops, to develop self trust. I pay a lot of attention to 'self trust' in the work that I do because it was a core challenge that I had to overcome on my path.

### Why is self trust so important?

Learning to trust yourself is incredibly important if you want to lose weight for good. When you trust yourself you will feel more confident and self assured. You will also be in a position to make more empowered decisions about your health and life.

No one knows you better than you do. Sure experts can share their insight, wisdom and experience but ultimately it is you that must decide what is right for you. You are the only one that has a deep and intimate all-knowing relationship with your body, mind, emotions and spirit. Losing weight for good involves cultivating the trust you have in yourself, so you can make decisions that are right for you.

### Developing your intuition.

A big part of learning to trust yourself is actively developing your own intuitive knowing. The more you tune in to your own intuition, the more you will be able to trust your own inner wisdom and strength. Listen to your intuition. Allow it to guide you to people that can inspire, encourage and show you how to become your own trusted source of information.

When you use your intuition, you can trust yourself to make healthy choices for yourself. It will also help you avoid the confusion and overwhelm that is so prevalent within the dieting and health arena.

**Allow your body to be your teacher.**

In my yoga retreats and classes, I always tell my students to allow their body to be their teacher and me to be their guide. If you are looking for other people to tell you how to live your life, you will always feel disconnected from your own inner wisdom and power.

The truth is that every-body is different. What is true for someone else may not be true for you. This is why it is critical that ultimately you become your own authority.

When experts make weight loss recommendations they will typically make them within their field of expertise. For example,

- Doctors recommend medication.
- Plastic surgeons recommend cosmetic procedures.
- Diet food companies recommend their 'low calorie' meals.
- Pharmaceutical companies recommend 'diet pills'.

Ask to be connected to the highest aspects of yourself and listen to your own body's wisdom. Pay close attention to the things that 'ring true' for you and trust yourself to know what is best for your own body.

Only you can decide what is right for you.

**Question everything.**

On your weight loss healing journey it is important that you learn to question everything.

Just the other day I read an excerpt out of a best-selling weight loss book by a medical doctor, saying that people can drink an unlimited number of diet drinks because they have 'no calories' in them.

Now I have to say that this personally does not ring true for me, because I know the harmful effects that regularly consuming any kind of fake food can have on the body. But rather than have me convince you of anything, ask your body and your own inner wisdom for answers.

As an experiment, drink a litre of 'diet soft drink' and then compare it to how you feel after drinking a litre of pure, filtered water. Your body always knows the truth.

## Learning to trust myself.

Early on in my weight loss journey I had real problems trusting myself. I was totally disconnected from my internal power and intuition and as a result I would habitually place all my trust in other people.

The trust issues that I encountered in those early days included valuing other peoples' opinions above my own, particularly the so called 'weight loss experts.'

I did not trust myself around food and would regularly binge eat in private. I followed restrictive diets whilst overriding the natural intuitive impulses of my body. I also found it difficult to trust compliments that other people would give me or in my ability to lose weight.

Looking back it was my lack of self trust that led me to incessantly override my body's inner wisdom. It was this approach to living, spread out over a number of years, which led to my health break down.

Something shifted in me the day my doctors recommended that I take a course of experimental medication. I knew the time had finally come for me to start trusting myself and in the process take back my power.

Although I didn't have all the answers at the time, I somehow knew that they would come to me when the time was right. And that is exactly what happened.

## Connect to your inner wisdom.

I believe that the best possible gift that I can give you is to help connect you to your own path, inner truth and personal power. From this place you will be best positioned to naturally restore your health and happiness in a way that is right for you.

When you have the courage to listen to yourself and trust in your inner wisdom, you will attract the right people and guidance to support your healing and growth. It is here that your greatest challenges will transform into your greatest opportunities.

---

# How to trust yourself.

Here are some ideas to help connect you to your inner wisdom:

- Start each day by asking to be connected to your higher self and inner knowing.

- Be childlike. Embody the qualities of innocence and wonder.

- Start small. Make unimportant, day-to-day decisions purely using your intuition and by tuning into your imagination.

- Pay attention to the natural rhythms of nature. Observe the flow of the seasons through trees, plants, birds, insects and animals.

- Do one thing that you have always wanted to do. Sign up for an art class, take a piano lesson or book that yoga retreat.

---

## Keep going until you succeed.

*"It doesn't matter if you try and try and try again, and fail. It does matter if you try and fail, and fail to try again."*

*~ Charles Kettering*

Your weight loss healing journey is exactly that, a journey. As on any journey there will be times when you will feel on path and other times when you feel as if you have gone off-track. The most important thing you can do is keep your gaze firmly fixed on your desired destination and just keep going until you succeed.

In the words of Thomas Edison, "I am not discouraged, because every wrong attempt discarded is another step forward."

## Failure leads to success.

I am someone who does not believe in the concept of failure. When we say that we have "failed" what we are really saying is that we have found a "strategy" that does not work for us.

It does not matter if you have tried and 'failed' to lose weight in the past. It also does not matter how long you have been struggling to lose weight, whether it is a few months, or a few decades. When you are ready to step into the light of self awareness, listen within, let go of the past, address and heal the real problem and do what is right for you. Your life will change for the better. In fact every area of your life will transform in miraculous ways.

Every time you try something there is an opportunity to learn something new. Each lesson helps you to experience new growth, gain new knowledge and move you in the direction of what you truly desire.

Try, fail, try, fail, try, fail, try, fail, try – SUCCEED!

## The power of persistence.

A child learns to walk by falling over many times before they finally figure out how to walk properly. Do you know that a child falls over approximately 700 times before they take their first step?

Do you try things a few times and then find yourself very quickly giving up? One way to tap into the power of persistence is to keep yourself inspired. Surround yourself with the inspiration and the support you need until you achieve the results you want.

Imagine if we had to learn to walk when we were 20 or 30 years old. I wonder if we would ever learn to walk. Imagine the things we would say: "Oh walking. I tried that a few times but I was useless."

Know that you do not need to reinvent the wheel. Getting the successful results that you desire is about modeling the strategies of people who have already created the results you desire.

If you do your inner healing work and start living in alignment with your truth, you will lose weight and get healthy very quickly. A healthy body and mind creates vibrant health.

This book is about revealing to you that weight loss is a healing journey. It is a road that I thankfully discovered quite by accident. It is a tried and true system for guaranteed permanent and natural weight loss.

## Bumps in the road.

Committing to losing weight for good doesn't mean that you won't hit any bumps along the path. Bumps are an essential part of the journey and will give you the opportunity to strengthen your mind as you progress.

The bumps in the road may push you off course or even slow you down. The important thing to realise is that, if you are committed to losing weight for good these bumps will pale in insignificance in comparison to what you will learn about yourself and the success that you will enjoy.

Any time you find yourself feeling challenged, just take some time out to reconnect with yourself. Spend time writing and journaling as well as doing the exercises in this book to gain a deeper understanding of who you are in the process of becoming.

## Challenges as opportunities in disguise.

Use weight loss as a chance to focus more on hope than fear, possibilities more than risks, options more than worry, the journey more than setbacks and opportunities more than challenges.

When you say that you are ready to do what it takes to heal and lose weight, what you are actually saying is that you want to address some things in your life.

Let the challenges that you experience spur you on to your weight loss success. I certainly wouldn't be the same woman that I am today without overcoming my own personal challenges.

Even if you slip up for a day or a week or a month, especially in the beginning, just know that this is normal. Slip ups do not matter as they are all part of the challenges you will encounter on your weight loss healing journey.

Just notice what else is going on around you and with as much kindness, love, consciousness and awareness as you can foster, simply get back up and keep moving towards your weight loss goals.

**Take it day by day.**

Just start by slowly making small changes in your habits and life so that you can allow the transformation to occur from within.

On your journey remember to keep things simple. Don't try and do everything all at once. Take your time and remember to be patient with yourself. Do what feels good to you and your body. Take small, baby steps and open yourself to embrace the concept of progress not perfection.

By bringing together the inner and outer aspects of healing your body, mind and emotions, you can lose weight. This is a holistic approach that will help you to heal yourself from the inside out.

Keep listening within to your true self and let your body and mind teach and support you as you move forward. When you make the inner changes with consciousness, your whole life will shift for the better.

# Afterword

*"A teacher of fear can't bring peace on Earth. We have been trying to do it that way for thousands of years. The person who turns inner violence around, the person who finds peace inside and lives it, is the one who teaches what true peace is. We are waiting for just one teacher. You're the one."*

*~ Byron Katie ~*

And now it is your turn. This is your opportunity to create your own weight loss healing journey filled with miracles, insights and opportunities for self discovery and personal growth.

Know that the road will not always be smooth. Let any bumps be an indication that you are on the right path. Whenever you need direction, simply look within. Ask for inner guidance to take you wherever you need to go, to find the answers that you desire.

When you take a natural approach to healing your body, mind and emotions by following the steps as outlined in this book, I know that you can change your body and your life, just like I did.

As you heal yourself you can break free of the dieting cycle of deprivation, restriction and frustration and start losing weight naturally and permanently.

I believe in you and I know that you can do it. I really look forward to one day having the pleasure of meeting you in person and hearing your personal weight loss success story.

# Additional Resources

**Katrina's Website:** www.KatrinaLoveSenn.com

**Documentaries**

'Super Size Me': www.MorganSpurlock.com

'Food Matters': www.FoodMatters.com

'Food Inc.': www.FoodIncMovie.com

'May I Be Frank?': www.MayIBeFrankMovie.com

'Fat, Sick and Nearly Dead': www.FatSickandNearlyDead.com

'The Tapping Solution': www.TheTappingSolution.com

'Simply Raw: Reverse Diabetes in 30 Days': www.Rawfor30Days.com

**Retreat Websites**

Skyros Holistic Retreat Centre: www.Skyros.com

The Hill That Breathes: www.TheHillThatBreathes.com

Sunflower Retreats: www.SunflowerRetreats.com

**Other Useful Health Information Websites**

Natural News: www.NaturalNews.com

Dr Mercola: www.Mercola.com

Dr Christine Northrup: www.DrNorthrup.com

Dr Rosy Daniel: www.HealthCreation.co.uk

# FREE eCourse
# 5 Steps to Transformation

If you would like to deepen your healing journey, please go to the following website and download your FREE eCourse called '5 Steps to Transformation'.

## www.StepsToTransformation.com

In the '5 Steps to Transformation' eCourse you will learn:

- How to feel powerful about your life right now, so that you can let go of the past and create a crystal clear vision for your future.

- How to identify and overcome unconscious blocks that may have stopped you in the past from achieving what you want.

- How to create a strong foundation for successful transformation in all areas of your life, even if you don't know where to start.

When you join you will receive Katrina's weekly newsletter which is filled with useful tips, ideas and inspiration for your healing journey.

It also includes the latest information on Katrina's upcoming programs, workshops and Yoga Retreats.

CPSIA information can be obtained at www.ICGtesting.com
Printed in the USA
LVOW07s2125010915

452395LV00002B/238/P